Professor Dame Elizabeth Nneka Anionwu is an Emeritus Professor of Nursing at the University of West London. In 1979, she set up the first ever UK sickle cell/thalassaemia nurse counselling service, based in Brent. She became a senior lecturer at the University College London's Institute of Child Health, was dean of the School of Adult Nursing Studies and Professor of Nursing at the University of West London (UWL), and also established the Mary Seacole Centre for Nursing Practice before her retirement in 2007.

She was vice-chairperson of the successful appeal for the Mary Seacole Memorial Statue that was unveiled in June 2016 and is now life patron of the Mary Seacole Trust. Elizabeth is also patron of the Sickle Cell Society and the Nigerian Nurses Charitable Association UK, and is vice-president of Unite Community Practitioners' and Health Visitors' Association (CPHVA). In 2018, Elizabeth was listed as one of the top seventy influential nurses and midwives between 1948 and 2018. In 2020, she was included in the top 100 Greatest Black Britons and as one of the fifty most influential BAME people in health. Elizabeth appeared in May 2020 as a guest on the BBC radio programme *Desert Island Discs*. In November 2020, she was included in the BBC 100 Women 2020 list and in 2021 the musician Dua Lipa dedicated her BRIT award to Elizabeth in recognition of her life-long fight against racial injustice and her advocacy for frontline workers.

DREAMS
FROM MY
MOTHER

Dame Elizabeth Anionwu

SEVEN DIALS

Originally published as *Mixed Blessings from a Cambridge Union* in
Great Britain in 2016 by ELIZAN Publishing
This revised and updated edition first published in
Great Britain in 2021 by Seven Dials,
an imprint of The Orion Publishing Group Ltd
Carmelite House, 50 Victoria Embankment
London EC4Y 0DZ

An Hachette UK Company

3 5 7 9 10 8 6 4 2

ISBN (Mass Market Paperback) 978 1 8418 8522 3
ISBN (eBook) 978 1 8418 8523 0
ISBN (Audio) 978 1 8418 8524 7

Printed and bound in Great Britain by Clays Ltd, Elcograf S.p.A.

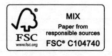

MIX
Paper from
responsible sources
FSC® C104740

www.orionbooks.co.uk

To my daughter, Azuka, my granddaughter, Rhianne, and my late parents

Contents

Foreword

I have been lucky enough to know Elizabeth Anionwu for a number of years. From the moment I met her, her intelligence, compassion and warmth shone forth. I know her as a patron of the Sickle Cell Society, an eminent nurse and professor and from when she was vice-chair of the Mary Seacole Memorial Statue Appeal. I have long admired her and her achievements, so I was more than happy to read her memoir, which provides a fascinating insight into her life and her dual-heritage Irish and Nigerian ancestry.

Elizabeth's memoir explores her early years, from her time spent in children's homes, to living with her mother then with her grandparents, and thereafter her life as an independent young woman. We are provided with an interesting insight into the social conventions and mores of the time when Elizabeth's mother was pregnant with her – in the late 1940s – and the reactions of family and the Church once Elizabeth, who is mixed race, was born.

Throughout the memoir, Elizabeth's mother's love and determination are clearly evident. And Elizabeth's first meeting and subsequent relationship with her Nigerian barrister father make for riveting reading.

Elizabeth's memoir illustrates her long and illustrious life, including her discovery and further research into the life of Mary Seacole, and her own efforts to improve the knowledge and treatment of sickle cell disease and thalassaemia.

There are very many gems in Elizabeth's reminiscences, including her comment to His Royal Highness the Prince of Wales during her investiture at Buckingham Palace, where she received her CBE. *Dreams from My Mother* is interwoven with Elizabeth's usual humour and insightfulness, and I very much enjoyed reading it.

—MALORIE BLACKMAN, OBE

Preface

My favourite photograph is a black and white one of me sitting on my mother's knee, possibly taken in 1948, the year after my birth. I don't know exactly how old I am – maybe between nine and fifteen months. She was coming to visit me at St Joan's Nursery, part of the Father Hudson's Care complex in Coleshill in Birmingham, where I'd been placed as the child of an unwed mother. You can actually see the home behind us; always with the windows open to let in the fresh, bracing air.

I think it tells an incredible story: I've got that afro – I love that head of hair on me – and I'm wrapped in a shawl. For a long time I couldn't work out what I was holding; I thought it looked like a toffee apple, but it's actually a rattle and one of my socks, which had fallen off. A friend pointed out to me (because I'm not very observant) that you can see my mum's chic bag lying on the bench. She's got that late forties style you see in films and looks very smart with her hair done.

I don't know who took the photo or its provenance. I don't know if it's the first picture she has of me. All the nuns of that era will be in their nineties or dead now, so they won't be able to tell me if it was an official photo or whether one of her friends took it. But what I really notice is how happy my mother looks. There's no stress in her face and she's got a little smile as she looks directly into the camera. Certainly no lowered eyes.

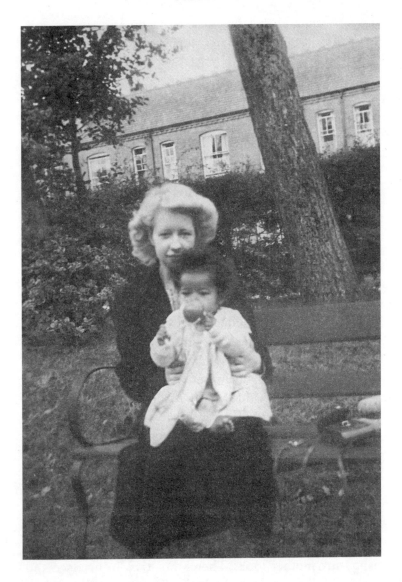

This photograph has had an impact on so many people. Many mixed-race people and parents of mixed-race children have commented on how proud my mum is – there is no shame or stigma in the photo in an era when it was virtually unheard of to have a brown-skinned child. Even just to see a photo of a white mother with her mixed-race child during that era is so uplifting, they say. I've had people come up to me after talks saying that it's this photo that resonates the most with them.

One person observed:

> You stand on the stage and talk about your life but, Elizabeth, you don't realise that you're talking about issues that many of us have felt the same way about. Black, white, being in two worlds, how society views people of mixed-race heritage – these are things some of us find it very difficult to talk about. I've learned a lot from your story and have taken away the words: 'For God's sake, be proud of who you are and stop being influenced by negative reactions within society.' I can see your pride and that you don't dwell on the negative things that have happened in your life. In other people's lives, they would be a two-hour lecture . . . but you just mention them and move on. Seeing how happy your mum looked, that's carried on through you.

Chapter 1:

A Golden Child

In 1945, my mother, aged nineteen, was the first in her family to go to university. If you look at it from the Irish-Catholic context, this was their time. People from Irish, Italian and Jewish backgrounds had fought for the British army in both wars and now wanted to make something of themselves, and education was the channel to do that.

The Charles Dickens quote from *Great Expectations* always goes through my mind: "'Which dear old Pip, old chap," said Joe, "you and me was ever friends. And when you're well enough to go out for a ride – what larks!"' That's the feeling I get from the family – the excitement they would have had telling the whole extended family about what my mother, Mary, had achieved – winning a scholarship to Cambridge University. And the effect it must have had on her. She would have been the toast of the family and everyone would have been so proud.

Her parents, Michael Furlong and Florence Sloan, had been first-generation immigrants born in Liverpool in 1896. They had grown up in the working-class Irish-Catholic dockland community then jokingly referred to as 'the capital of Ireland'. My mother, Mary Furlong, was born on 10 October 1926 at home on Lindsay Road in Walton. As her grandmother and aunt were also called Mary, she was given the pet name of Maureen, Gaelic for 'Little Mary'.

From the age of three, Mary pestered her father to read the newspaper each day. 'She was mad about learning to read and she nagged your grandfather. Every time he picked up a book she asked him what the words meant, so in the end he sat her down and taught her to read,' my half-sister Marion once told me. As a consequence, she was able to read and write when she started primary school.

My grandfather had come from a family that embraced education despite many obstacles. In the nineteenth century, at a time when schooling for non-Anglican children was illegal in Ireland, his maternal grandfather, Michael Kehoe, had been a 'hedge schoolmaster' in Wexford County, teaching Catholic children in out-of-the-way places such as quiet roadsides to avoid detection. If caught, he could have been imprisoned, executed or transported – so he hid his teaching books on a shelf up the wide chimney. His Latin primer book was passed down to my great-aunt Kate, who became a teacher, but 'it was dried up and fell apart'.

When his daughter Mary Kehoe moved to England around 1871, she took up domestic work and had a great desire to have all of her children properly educated, explained Kate. Thanks to her determination, my grandfather – the youngest of seven surviving children – became one of the first scholarship boys to attend the fee-paying Catholic Institute in Liverpool.

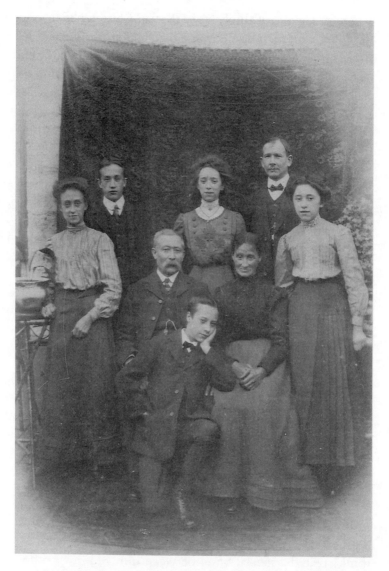

My Furlong great-grandparents in 1914. Grandad, aged fourteen, is kneeling.

There's a legendary family story that on a Sunday afternoon, he failed to return home immediately after performing his duties as an altar boy at the Benediction. His mother went out looking for him and was so incensed to find him in an Italian ice-cream parlour, she hauled him out by the ear. The impact of Catholicism on the Furlong family passed down to the next generation, as my aunt Sheila and a cousin of my mother would eventually become nuns.

When the First World War broke out in 1914, my grandfather, aged eighteen, enlisted in an Irish regiment, the Connaught Rangers. My mother later told me his regiment had a reputation for marksmanship and, inspired by this tradition, he became a crack shot. He regretted this later, when it led to his being selected for a firing squad, which had to execute cowards and deserters. On his return home after the war, he took a civil service examination that qualified him to enter Customs and Excise. In 1924, he married her mother, Florence, who had been working as a bookkeeper.

After my mother was born two years into their marriage, there followed three more children: a son, Michael, in 1928, then, nearly a decade later, two more daughters: Sheila was born in 1935 and Pat in 1937. My grandfather was an incredibly intelligent man and head of the household; my grandmother doted on him. Every morning there was a ritual where she would whip him up a disgusting concoction of raw eggs in milk, setting it in front him before he drank it back and left for work. I always remember his lovely trilby and that he was a bit of a chain-smoker, with a pipe and cigarettes. He was also very bookish, which I think created a special bond between him and my mother.

My mother described the early years of her parents' marriage in a letter to me:

[As my father] was moved from one temporary post to another, they stayed in boarding houses. I was born during this period, and travelled about with them. When I was two, my father was given a permanent post in Stafford, which was then a sleepy little market town, very English, conservative and Protestant. I don't think he ever felt much at home there.

He was a member of the Fabian Society, the avant-garde of socialism in those days, an ardent Catholic and still interested in Irish politics, sympathising with the Republican movement. Religion and politics were frequently talked about in our house, and although I didn't understand much of it, I formed a strong impression that my father was a fish out of water among his colleagues and acquaintances.

The rented house in Stafford where the family finally settled was a spacious three-storey family home in a leafy cul-de-sac and a world away from transient boarding houses and uncertainty that had come before. It had three bedrooms, a couple of attic rooms and a front and back garden. There was an elderberry bush and an apple tree, which the local children were free to come and take fruit from. Neighbours living in nearby semi-detached houses in this middle-class area of Stafford included the owner of two coal mines and a prison parson.

My grandmother was often very poorly (she was later diagnosed with pernicious anaemia – essentially a deficiency of vitamin B12), but what I really remember about her was her lovely smile, great sense of humour and huge belly laugh. She reminded me of the Queen Mother because she was short, plump and – until she got older – very jovial.

She also loved storytelling; the impact of Irish culture was so much more obvious in my grandmother. She'd spent her early life in Ireland but had grown up with her extended family in Liverpool, which was an Irish-Catholic enclave. She was a devout Catholic and, while she was very humorous, she was also very narrow-minded.

The most insightful description of her was from my mother in a letter: 'Two things stand out in my mind about my mother. First, her devotion to the Catholic faith, the obverse of which was a somewhat bigoted attitude to other denominations. Secondly, her poor health, which seemed to decline as the size of the family increased.'

However, even with two much younger sisters and a mother who was often ill, Mary wasn't expected to take on household chores. She wasn't necessarily 'the favoured one', but she was obviously a gifted child and there was a lot of hope, expectation and love poured into my mother. I think she was probably spoiled a little because of it. I don't know for sure, but she was certainly given a lot of attention. Both of her parents recognised her potential and, while she seemed closer to my grandfather, I'm sure her mother was still proud of her. It was clear both of them recognised her academic abilities, and she was treated slightly differently as a result.

Her younger sister Pat gives the impression that my mother was slightly self-centred with her siblings, leaving them in awe of their older sister – or she was at least someone they'd have to negotiate around. Pat remembers: 'I used to get your mum to do my Latin homework because I was no good at it and I would clean her bike in exchange because she wouldn't do it for nothing.' Sheila was very sporty and won all sorts of cups and medals for the school and Pat, who excelled at maths instead of Latin and sports, used to be irritated by the teachers comparing her to her sisters.

Living in Stafford during the Second World War, Mary was a typical teenager, frustrated and irritated by the every-day privations and food shortages: 'We lived in a safe area, so I can't pretend that the tragedies and triumphs of the Second World War made much impression on me. I remember the civilian inconveniences; gas masks, rationing, having to share the school with evacuees, the blackout and the sudden disappearance of organised amusement for my age group.'

But even war and its effect on society didn't hold her back from success. Attending the local convent school, Mary stayed on to take the Higher School Certificate – the equivalent of the later A levels – then won a scholarship to Newnham College, Cambridge, to read Classics, during the last year of the war. It was at Cambridge where my mother would meet my father.

Chapter 2:

Cambridge Life

Around the time my mother won her place at Cambridge, there had been a host of educational reforms opening up universities to women – Cambridge awarded their first degree to a woman in 1948, the last of the big-name UK institutions to do so.[1] My mother was in the position to take advantage of it all. As a bright woman with a loving family and good free schooling, all the factors were coming together for the first time.

I think Cambridge must have been beautiful for her. She walked into a privileged society – a learning environment of the first degree, which she must have found so joyous because she loved her Classics and her books. A women-only college, Newnham actively encouraged female students from all social classes.[2] I don't know anyone who went to Cambridge with her and she never spoke about it later in her life, but if you're very gifted and you're doing things that nobody else in your family is able to do, then surely that gives you confidence? Gaining admission in spite of the deprivations of war and all the restrictions, that would have given her a real sense of achievement.

She would also have enjoyed the social side of university life (after all, she had me). She liked dressing up, she liked lipstick and going out dancing. On the one hand, my mother was a real intellectual character and, on the other, she enjoyed life. She obviously flourished. At Cambridge, she won the Goodhart Memorial Prize for Classics in 1945 and the Eleanor Purdie Prize for Greek in 1946, and she gained a First in her Classics prelim exams. The Newnham College authorities later told my grandfather that she was expected to obtain a First in part one of her tripos.

While she was excelling in the academic world, I know from my own health visitor background that the brightest of people sometimes don't have any idea about sex. My mother wouldn't have had sex education at school and the war meant she'd had a very sheltered upbringing, without even the normal opportunities to socialise with other teenagers. Nobody would have explained that there's a logical process to sex and pregnancy, or even mentioned the passions of life. Her entire world would have been education, religion and home life. She would simply have moved from Stafford to Cambridge. And it's this bit that I wonder about. When did she start socialising? When did she start mixing with men? When did she meet my father? When did sexual activities first occur?

My mother became pregnant with me in her second year of university, in November 1946. This was one of the worst things she could do as a woman. In that era, and from an Irish-Catholic family, to become pregnant as an unmarried woman was a disaster. Once my mother realised she was pregnant, she couldn't bring herself to tell her parents the truth. I can't help but think about the relationship she had with her father – she wouldn't have wanted his bubble of expectation, adoration and love to burst. My grandfather was an intelligent man and had won his scholarship to school, so she was really following in his footsteps and that must have created such a special bond. It makes it all the more sad and poignant for it to have come crashing down.

It must have been terrible. That's before you take into account all of the expectations of her family. I often wonder what she must have gone through mentally the minute she missed her period. What was she going to do? Did she go into denial? I don't know any of her friendship circles, so would she have revealed it to anybody? There would have been fear, but I think shame would have been the biggest factor.

All the things affecting this situation: religion, class and the aspiration to move up in the world, education (which was really important to the Furlong family and its history) and (what her parents didn't know about at this point) race; you have the family thinking she's doing well, winning prizes in her first and second years — but what was it like for her as her abdomen expanded? After all, she was small like me, not even five feet tall, so she would easily be showing.

In the end, it was when she went home in the spring of 1947, when she would have been around six months pregnant, that my grandmother realised what had happened. 'Mum was making Mary a summer skirt and when she went to try it on her, it didn't fit on the waist,' my auntie Pat told me. 'Mum asked her if she was pregnant and she replied, "Yes." Mum said: "When were you going to tell me about it?" Mary replied, "I wasn't. I was going to go and jump off a bridge."'

Chapter 3:

The Dossier

Letter from my mother, 18 April 1994:

My parents' reaction to the news of my pregnancy was sheer horror. They insisted that it must be kept secret, and I was virtually a prisoner in the house until I could be sent to a home for unmarried mothers, run by nuns in Birmingham. The official story was that I had had a nervous breakdown, and gone to stay with relatives in Ireland to recuperate.

Shock and silence surrounded everything. My aunts were twelve and ten at the time and weren't told anything about me, while my uncle Michael was away at sea. My grandfather might have written to him, as they had a very loving relationship but, to this day, I don't know for sure. Looking at the Irish and Catholic narratives around illegitimacy – never mind mixed-race issues – silence, shame and stigma suffocated everything surrounding my arrival.

The stigma of being an unwed mother in 1947 was insurmountable. From the Victorians' 'fallen women' to the British workhouses for unmarried mothers (the last of which were closed in the 1930s),[1] giving birth to a child out of wedlock had many connotations, including being morally lax and mentally unwell. From 1913 to 1959, a girl's family could use the Mental Deficiency Act[2] to label pregnant unwed women under twenty-one as moral imbeciles and send them to asylums. This was also in the aftermath of the Second World War, when a woman had a duty to help rebuild the country by being a good wife and mother – a country struggling with the fact of its 70,000 illegitimate children born to American servicemen.

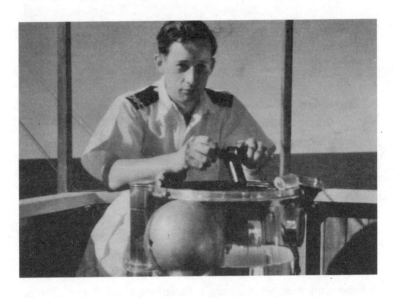

Uncle Michael.

Even as I got older, there was so much silence around my birth; I never wanted to ask my mother questions about sensitive issues because my stepfather and half-brothers and -sisters were always around when I went to see her. She did respond to some letters in March 1972 and 1994, when I asked her direct questions about my father and her life, but even they weren't always the full story – her lived experience was different from the stories I'd hear from Auntie Pat or my own understanding.

In 2011, eight years after my mother's death, and at the grand age of sixty-four, I at last decided to do something about what had been at the back of my mind for decades. I only had the one photo of myself from my childhood, but I could also remember a tiny one of me as a toddler riding a tricycle in the hall, which I could no longer find. So I decided to find out if there were any photos of me during my years at Nazareth House.

After getting in touch with The Sisters of Nazareth Archive at Nazareth House in Hammersmith, they advised that I contact Father Hudson's Care in Birmingham. Now a Catholic social care agency helping older people, people with care needs, families and children, this was where I'd lived as a baby until the age of three and a half.

While they now no longer deal with child adoption, they realised that many people wanted to connect with their own beginnings and find a sense of identity. In 1993, they set up the Origins department with 40,000 records on the children who had been adopted within their organisation dating back to 1902.[3] After they recommended that I send a letter with my details, I was called by their social worker, Siobhán. Much to my disappointment, she told me that no photographs existed. However, what they did have was correspondence about my time living there and at Nazareth House.

She asked if I wanted to come and visit her, as her offices were in Coleshill in the same place where I would have spent the first years of my life. It felt so exciting and a little weird and incongruous to go back there. But rather than emotion, it was my curiosity and love of history that powered my interest in visiting. Looking around and realising this was where my mum would have come to see me was an incredible feeling.

In her office, Siobhán handed me a thick blue dossier with my name on the front. It contained fifty-seven documents – from a crisp, new birth certificate (a sharp contrast to the tatty, torn and Sellotaped copy that my mother had given me in 1965) to a neat list of Mother's visits. There was also letter after letter written by my mother and grandfather to the Reverend (later Canon) Flint, who was the administrator of Father Hudson's Care and secretary of the Birmingham Diocesan Rescue Society.

Dating from April 1947, a few months before my birth in July, to September 1956, when I left Nazareth House Convent aged nine, these records were a historian's dream. I was amazed by both them and the fact that the dossier was mine to take away.

Back at home on my own – I couldn't be around anyone else – I started to read its contents. Siobhán had prepared a letter that explained what was inside:

Dear Elizabeth,

We were first contacted by your maternal grandparents when your mother was pregnant. We understood that your mother, Mary Furlong, was a student at Cambridge University who had completed two years studying Classics. She had become pregnant and as she was just beginning to show, her parents were keen to have Mary provided with accommodation so as to conceal the pregnancy. Adoption was mentioned as the plan. At this time, we were advised that your father's name was unknown. It is probable that at this stage Mary's parents assumed he was white.

Ploughing through the letters inside was so moving. My mother's and grandfather's words felt like a window into the world before I was born. The thought that struck me was: *My God, the date of this letter shows that my mum would have been eight months pregnant and she's about to have me*; I'd never experienced such a thing before. The correspondence was an insight into the emotional impact that my birth had had on such a devout Catholic family.

Chapter 4:

Uncovering History

With my mother in the later stages of pregnancy, the letters showed that her parents recovered from the initial shock and quickly moved into action. The plan was that my grandmother would take me in as her own so my mother could return to Cambridge and carry on with her education.

The big concern was the fact they needed to hide Mary away from the prying eyes of the local community before the birth, so they turned to the Church for help. It would have been their parish priest, Father Cregg, who I believe was in the diocese in Stafford and a friend of my grandfather's, who would have put them in contact with Reverend Flint.

Letter from my grandfather to Reverend Flint, 22 April 1947:

Many thanks for your letter of the 18th inst. stating that you have arranged temporary accommodation for Mary. If it is at all possible, I would be extremely obliged if the good people who are to afford Mary accommodation could be in a position to let her stay on the day that she visits them, subject of course to their being fully satisfied in every respect.

Mary is beginning to show and, the distance to the

Railway Station being fairly lengthy, we do not want her to come under any possible scrutiny of neighbours that can be avoided. Subject to your ratification, I suggest that when Mary travels to Birmingham she takes sufficient clothing with her to enable her to stay with the people offering the accommodation and thus prevent her having to make the second journey. Any further clothing or items that she may require could be sent on later and in the event of the people in Birmingham not wanting to put Mary up, which please God will not occur, I would bring the suitcase back with me.

These letters are short and to the point, but behind their formality is a sense of urgency that reveals the fears, challenges, stigma and turmoil facing my mother and my family. It also reveals the administrative hurdles and delays encountered in finding a nursery cot for me during 1947 – the start of the post-war baby boom with one million births in Britain that year alone.[1]

My grandfather took the lead in organising everything, demonstrating the loving relationship he had with my mother and the fact that he and my grandmother wanted to help and protect her – there's never any sense of condemnation. So, with Reverend Flint's help, my mother went to live with a Birmingham family for a few weeks until her place at the mother-and-baby home became available.

It was Siobhán, the Father Hudson Care Origins social worker, who pointed out to me that this was not at all typical of this time. Because my family were devout and middle class, with status within their community, the news of an illegitimate child would reflect badly not only on them but also on the Church; and so this was a family the authorities wanted to protect and rally round.

The letters also illustrate the substantial level of advice and financial support offered by the Church to encourage my mother's return to her studies. Comparing it to well-known stories from around that time such as Philomena Lee, an Irish unwed mother who was forced to give up her son for adoption by nuns in 1952,[2] it seems a pretty unique situation. The Church was advising via respectful communication; there were no diktats for now. If my mother had come from a different background, she might have found things much more difficult and, in turn, my start in life could have been much worse.

But, even with the best will in the world, it's obvious that everyone involved was feeling the strain, and towards the end of April their anxiety is palpable, as it became clear that my mother was beginning to think about getting a job rather than going back to Cambridge. While her parents were prepared to support her decision to keep her baby, they were less happy in the matter of her education and called upon Reverend Flint to help her see sense. Letter from my grandfather to Reverend Flint, 30 April 1947:

Her mother has tried to reason her into accepting the situation as she, her mother sees it, namely that it would be better for her to go back to Cambridge, finish her course, and thus be [able] to obtain a better position and so enable her to provide better still for the baby . . . If you are in agreement with the idea that it would be better for Mary to return to Cambridge when the first term of next year commences, I would esteem it a favour if you would use your influence to get her to see that such a course would in the long run be better for herself and her offspring.

Alongside this contentious subject, my mother's ration book took centre stage. Two years after the war, rationing was still widespread in Britain to help counter food, clothing, soap and fuel shortages.[3] It seems that the extra clothing coupons needed for the baby's layette were threatening to bring her pregnancy out into the open. Letter from my grandfather to Reverend Flint, 14 May 1947:

I have had a letter from Mary in which she told me of her visit and of your kindness and help in the matter of the ration book difficulty. Mrs Furlong has asked me to express her gratitude to you for your help in this matter as it has been a source of great worry to her, as it appeared to be an obstacle that we could not overcome and was likely to nullify all the efforts which had been made to keep the matter away from local knowledge.

I am also very much obliged for your talk to Mary on her future and your promised assistance in the matter of the child. We had a very sympathetic letter from the Tutor at Newnham College and one was also written by her to Mary. This letter, coupled with your assistance in the matter, will, I feel sure, be sufficient to induce Mary to change her viewpoint and persuade her that her best course is to resume her studies at Cambridge at the commencement of the next year's course.

At the end of May, my mother moved into the mother-and-baby home, somewhat earlier than planned. Three weeks later, the precious clothing coupons finally arrived, just two weeks before my birth.

MEMO
50 Board of Trade clothing coupons
sent to Mary Furlong on 17 June 1947

Then on 2 July 1947, I was born at Loveday Street Maternity Hospital in Birmingham. I was discharged with my mother back to the mother and baby home where, nine days later, I was baptised in the chapel.

When my grandparents came to visit, they were greeted by one of the home's Irish nuns. Walking down the corridor to my mother's room, she turned and said: 'To be sure, the baby's a little dark.' As my auntie Pat later drily commented: 'That put the kibosh on bringing you back home because you would have been the only coloured kid in Stafford.' It would take a further two months before my mother would reveal the name of my father to the nuns.

Chapter 5:
Hard Times

All the wheels that had been set in motion came crashing to a stop when it became apparent I had a Black father. Until 1918, it's estimated there were around 20,000–30,000 Black people living in Britain, including seaman and soldiers based in cities such as London, Liverpool, Bristol and Glasgow, along with students like my father from Africa and the Caribbean.[1] In the Second World War, this number grew to 150,000 with the arrival of the US Army and other Black workers from the Caribbean and West Indies. More than 12,000 West Indians served in the British forces during the war, including the Royal Air Force and the Women's Auxiliary Air Force.[2]

Many Britons were shocked by the segregation laws of the US and welcomed the American Black GIs who were often politer and kinder than their brash white counterparts. But there was still widespread prejudice and racism: in 1942, the Home Secretary, Herbert Morrison, informed the war cabinet that 'some British women appear to find a peculiar fascination in associating with men of colour', while women who dated Black GIs were considered 'a very loose and undesirable sort of person'.

In the 2019 book *Britain's 'Brown Babies'*, Professor Lucy Bland explores the stories of the 2,000 mixed-race babies who were born to Black GIs and British white women. All of these children were labelled as illegitimate because the US Army refused the Black GIs permission to marry under the argument that thirty of the then forty-eight US states had anti-miscegenation laws. Just under half were placed in children's homes or fostered, as adoption agencies considered it too difficult to place mixed-race children. Prejudice and racism blighted the lives of those who stayed with their parents and their illegitimacy added another layer of shame.[3]

As Auntie Pat commented: 'There might have been a few more [mixed-race babies] because we did have American troops during the war, but your mum couldn't possibly have said you were hers. Anyhow, the parish priest said the gossip would be so bad and that it would have a very bad effect on the family.' Father Cregg advised my family that they could no longer bring me home. Even though my grandmother still wanted to adopt me, the priest believed the truth would get out that I was my mother's child.

Thinking back now and knowing that both my mother and grandmother wanted to keep me, I can't help but think that the Church doesn't sound very caring. It's about protecting its image through a respectable Catholic family. They didn't want anything to be revealed in the local parish that could besmirch their status. It wasn't coming from the family themselves.

Soon, adoption was proposed as a possible solution. However, in a letter from my mother in 1994, she explained: 'My parents had impressed on me that I could not keep the baby at home, and wanted me to have her adopted. This was against my wishes, and it was a relief to me when the nuns put an end to the argument, telling us categorically that there was no chance of finding adoptive parents for a coloured child. (It must be remembered that this was over forty-five years ago, when a half-caste child in provincial England was a rare phenomenon.)

My mother's obstinate nature also came to the surface when she announced she wanted to call me Artemis, after the Greek goddess of the hunt. This was firmly vetoed by my grandmother (I can imagine the row), so instead I was baptised Elizabeth Mary Furlong, having been born on the Catholic feast day celebrating the Visitation of the Blessed Virgin Mary to her cousin Elizabeth.

The strain of events began to affect all of those involved and it became apparent that I would have to be placed in a home. Letter from my grandfather to Reverend Flint, 5 August 1947:

> . . . I saw Mary on Sunday last on my visit to Francis Way and she appeared to be in a very low state, and I think that she will need a holiday of a bracing nature before she will be fit to resume at Newnham. Mrs Furlong is not keeping too grand and will be going for a short holiday at the end of August. In these circumstances, I am writing to ask if it is possible for you to say when Mary's child will be accepted into the Home and Mary be permitted to return to Stafford.
>
> I understand from Mary that you have a waiting list and I thus appreciate that the situation is difficult, but, if it is possible for an early admittance of Mary's child to be allowed, it would facilitate matters greatly for me and would allow Mary to accompany her Mother on holiday and to get herself fit to resume her studies at Cambridge in October. If it will be of any assistance, or if you so desire it, either Mrs Furlong or myself will willingly come over to Coleshill to see you.

Hoping that you do not consider this letter presumptuous, and thanking you for all you have done for us to date . . .

Alongside the worry of finding me a place in a home, my mother still hadn't given any details to anyone about my father. They knew he wasn't white, that was for sure. She was also trying to decide whether to return to her studies, the option desired by her family and the Catholic clergy.

At the end of August 1947, two months after my birth, my mother told the nuns my father's name: Lawrence Ani-onwu, aged twenty-four, single, a student at Cambridge from Nigeria. She didn't reveal his identity to me until my request to her in 1972, when I was twenty-four years old myself.

Chapter 6:
Mother-and-Baby

My mother and I spent six months together in the mother-and-baby home – Siobhán, the Origins social worker, commented in her letter to me: 'it was usual for mothers to spend around three months there with their babies.'

I know from my own training as a nurse and health visitor just how important this length of time would have been for both of us. Part of our curriculum centred on the work of British psychiatrist John Bowlby, who concluded in 1951 that 'to grow up mentally healthy the infant and young child should experience a warm, intimate and continuous relationship with his mother (or permanent mother substitute) in which both find satisfaction and enjoyment'.[1] The BBC also made some incredible films that we were shown on our course, demonstrating the impact of separation of children and their failure to thrive as a result of mourning their mother.

Looking back on what was the norm in the 1940s, as long as the child was fed, clothed and kept warm, this was considered adequate care. There wasn't even the understanding that a constant change of carers in a children's home or via fostering would cause confusion for a child. I often think watching documentaries such as *Long Lost Family*, about people who have been separated from their mothers, that you can see the trauma and impact it's had on their lives;

I think it often stops them from trusting and making relationships with others. Stories from Irish unwed mothers and their children at the Magdalene laundries and the industrial schools who were separated and incarcerated by the Church for years show the damage that was done.[2]

Until I got those records in 2011, I had it in my mind I had been in the mother-and-baby home for three months, so I was genuinely surprised and amazed that we'd had such a long time together. It also gave me another bit of information as to why life turned out all right for me in terms of my psychological state. Just the physicality of washing me and clothing me and playing with me – my mother would have been responsible for all that. We know the incredible relationship most mothers have with their babies in those first six months – they're so dependent. My mother was there and was a constant figure for a defenceless child. Thinking of my own daughter, it's such a lovely period because it's before they get feisty when you're feeding, changing and putting them to sleep.

It also strikes me how much more difficult it would have been for my mum to hand me over and place me in a children's home. But they didn't know any better and what was the alternative? She couldn't take me home because she was worried about the negative impact it would have had on the reputations of her family and her two younger sisters. I know I was lucky to have those six months, however difficult it would have been for her watching me grow from this baby to a plump, sitting, six-month-old baby. That's huge. What she went through would resonate with all mothers.

Then there was the suddenness of these decisions: when the time finally came for us to be parted, she was given just three days' notice. Letter to Mother Dolores, 19 December 1947:

Dear Mother Dolores, re Baby Furlong

Miss Furlong may arrange to bring her baby to Coleshill on Monday next, 22nd inst. if it is convenient for you to discharge her.

Yours sincerely

Administrator WF/mf

I was to be placed in St Joan's Nursery, part of the Father Hudson's Care complex in Coleshill, while my mother would return home to her parents in Stafford. It was three days before Christmas in 1947.

Chapter 7:

New Lives

God knows what that Christmas was like for my mother. They were a Catholic family so they'd have been going to church, but she must have been very lonely in herself and missing me. She couldn't even have spoken about me in the house, as her younger sisters knew nothing about my arrival. In 1994, later on in her life, my mother wrote me a letter about her life around this time:

I went home to Stafford, as there seemed no immediate alternative. I deferred to my parents' wishes by telling nobody of Elizabeth's existence, but I refused to go back to college. I didn't want to be parted from Elizabeth indefinitely, and the sort of academic career that I had hoped for simply would not have been open to a woman with an illegitimate child. The climate of opinion in such matters was very different in those days from what it is now.

I took a sketchy course at a business college, and got a job in a local office. It paid for my board at home, and the fees at Father Hudson's, but my aim was to find employment that would get me away from home and into a more freethinking atmosphere. Shorthand, which I was good at, seemed to offer a possible stepping stone to work as a journalist, and I went to advanced classes in the evenings.

My mother's decision not to continue with her studies must have come as a bombshell and a deep disappointment to both her parents and the Church; indeed, Reverend Flint had offered to waive the nursery fees to make it easier for her to return to Cambridge. I can imagine the horror of all the key players who had genuinely pulled out all the stops to encourage my mother to complete her studies.

Although she says she gave up Cambridge because she couldn't foresee a career with everything that had happened, I can't believe she wouldn't have been incredibly sad and disappointed. The fact she referred to her mother as 'narrow-minded' and she had been to Cambridge where she would have been exposed to much wider thoughts and discussions, plus the fact she didn't have me with her would have contributed to these feelings. The contrast must have been huge. There were so many secrets and lies, and I think the only escape for her was in her books.

My auntie Pat recalls: 'She was always reading and she switched off when she read. [I remember] she was in our sitting room downstairs in the big armchair with her legs curled up underneath her, which was where she liked to sit, and she was reading a book and I was sitting at the table doing homework. She put her hand round and said something to me which I didn't understand, because she was asking me in Greek for the Greek dictionary on the sideboard.'

She was obviously living the language and my mother would have come out of her zone and realised she needed to talk in English – it makes me wonder about the worlds that she lived in.

Ultimately, though, I think she didn't want to be in anyone's debt anymore and felt an incredible degree of responsibility towards me; and you can see her fiery, individualistic self-worth in this decision. She got herself into this situation and she was going to get herself out of it. She had no intention of letting go of me, either – she was retaining that link. She firmly but politely thanked Reverend Flint for all of his support one week after she handed me over:

Stafford, 30 December 1947
Dear Revd Father,
  Would you please let me know when it will be convenient for me to come and visit Elizabeth, and what the usual arrangements are about visiting? If there is anything that Elizabeth needs in the way of clothes, perhaps you would send me her clothing coupons, and I will buy the necessary articles, and bring them with me to Coleshill when I come.
  I appreciate very much your offer to look after Elizabeth without payment in order to allow me to continue my studies at Cambridge, but after thinking it over carefully, I have decided not to return to college. I am hoping to obtain a post shortly, and I shall then be able to pay for the child's maintenance. In the meantime, my father is willing to accept responsibility for payment. Will you please let me know what arrangement in this matter will suit you?
  I would like to thank you very much for all that you have done for Elizabeth and for myself. My parents and I are deeply grateful to you.

A few days later, she received a response. I was staggered to read it – she had to wait so long before she was allowed to see me. Letter from the home's administrator, 2 January 1948:

. . . normal visiting days are the first and third Sundays of the month from two to four, but if Sunday travel is difficult for you I could arrange for any afternoon suitable to you if you will kindly let me know.

The idea my mother could only visit me twice a month for two hours seems so horrible. Even though I know the context of the time in the late 1940s, I don't understand why my mother wasn't allowed to visit more frequently – maybe she couldn't even afford to – but it just comes across as so rigid. Today, it's understandably seen as harsh and cruel, and it's clear to me that they didn't know the harm that could come about to both mothers and babies experiencing these extended periods of separation.

When you think of all the things the Church did to support my mother and grandparents, I can't believe it was done deliberately. The only thing it does make me think of is the Catholic Church's attitude towards other unmarried mothers: they needed to be punished for their sins and there was no responsibility on people to be kind to them. But then that doesn't come out in my mother's story. A good example is what happened when children were admitted to hospital around this time – you couldn't just go and visit them. You had to request a pass and go during strict visiting hours. Babies would be kept in cots behind glass windows because the hospital was more worried about infection than the psychological support for the parents and children.

So my mother was issued with a pass that enabled her to visit me at the nursery for the first time on Saturday, 10 January 1948. She next wanted to visit on Wednesday, 11 February. I'm curious to know why a whole month had elapsed, but whatever the reason, my mother's self-reliant spirit shines through. Letter to Reverend Flint, 2 February 1948:

I am sorry that I have not been able to pay anything towards Elizabeth's maintenance. I have not yet obtained a post, as I am taking a three months' business course in order to qualify for a secretarial position. As you know, my father has offered to take entire responsibility for the child, but I am extremely reluctant to accept this offer. I feel that it is my own responsibility. I think you will understand my feelings on this point.

I would like to thank you very much for all that you have done for Elizabeth. I hope that it will not be long before I can arrange to have her with me and look after her myself, but in the meantime, I know she is in the best possible hands.

These worlds show the pangs of separation that must have affected my mother. It must have been incredibly sad – and more disappointment was to follow. Letter from the home's administrator, 5 February 1948:

Dear Miss Furlong,

Thank you for your letter received this morning. Unfortunately, I cannot enclose a visiting pass as, due to a recent outbreak of diphtheria, the Doctor has forbidden all visiting for the time being. Elizabeth is very well and I am hoping that we shall get no more than the three cases now in isolation.

The letter went on to reassure my mother that maintenance fees would be withheld until she started work. She replied by return that she would like to come as soon as visiting recommenced – but astonishingly, nearly two months later, she wrote to Reverend Flint pointing out that she had not heard anything about her request for a pass, or the outcome of the diphtheria outbreak. She asked permission to visit me on Wednesday, 31 March. This would make it nearly three months since she had been able to see me.

After this, letters are fewer and further between. There is a request from Reverend Flint to see my mother when she visits me, although the topic for discussion isn't revealed. In August 1948, she writes to him announcing that she has commenced work and can now start to pay for my maintenance.

Then on 3 September, it is my mother who makes a request to see Reverend Flint. Judging from a letter she writes on 23 October, I believe the subject of this meeting to have been my father. In the letter, my mother informs Reverend Flint that she will be seeing my father on Saturday, 30 October and requests a pass for him to accompany her on a visit to see me. That is (she adds), assuming that Reverend Flint will have no objection. I am nearly sixteen months old and presume that this will be my father's first sight of me.

23 October 1948
Dear Revd Father,

You may remember that, on the occasion of my visit to Coleshill about two months ago, we had some conversation on the subject of Elizabeth's father.

I received a letter from him today, saying that he will be in Birmingham next Saturday, 30 October. I am arranging to meet him on that date, and would like to bring him to see Elizabeth.

We have not yet reached any definite decision about our future plans, as I personally find it impossible to discuss such a question in letters, and I imagine that Laurie has the same difficulty.

I hope, however, that we shall reach some clear understanding when we meet next Saturday. I agree that it would be foolish to continue the acquaintance if it is not to lead to marriage.

However, I trust that you will have no objection to Laurie's coming with me to visit Elizabeth on this occasion.

What happened when they visited me remains a mystery, as my mother and I never fully talked about it. In addition to this letter, there is an undated note from Reverend Flint to the nursery revealing my mother's hope of marriage, plans to return to Africa with my father and that my grandparents were in agreement. And somewhere in my memory is a recollection of being told that my father had visited me as a baby. But reading this note in 2011 was the first time I became aware that my parents had planned to marry and return to Nigeria together.

Looking at my favourite photograph of me sitting on my mother's knee, I wonder whether it could have been taken by my father. After all, he was a well-off Nigerian student studying at college, so the chances of him having a camera are high; he would have had the resources and inclination to keep memories of that. I know they wrote to each other – did he send her the photo that would bring my life so much joy?

On 11 December, enquiring about an illness in the nursery, my mother asked when visiting was likely to be resumed. Once again, it meant another Christmas apart, and she asked whether it would be possible to visit me on Boxing Day, but the reply was in the negative.

13 December 1948
Dear Miss Furlong,

Thank you for your letter received this morning. Elizabeth is quite well, though we have had further cases of whooping cough among the young babies who were in more immediate contact with the original cases.

I am hoping that it will not spread to Elizabeth's side of the nursery and of course we are taking every precaution.

As we do not know yet the full extent of our troubles, I am afraid I cannot give a definite date as to when visiting will be resumed, but I am certain that we shall not be able to start visits again by Boxing Day.

With all best wishes.
Yours sincerely
Administrator WF/mf

The outbreak of whooping cough was to linger for several months. My mother was informed in February 1949 that I had caught it, and seemingly badly enough to warrant being able to visit me without restrictions. Letter from the home's administrator, 2 February 1949:

I am sorry to have to inform you that Elizabeth has contracted the whooping cough and is having rather severe spasms. If you would like to visit her, you may come at any time.

Further visits are recorded in April and May. In July, my mother wrote to (now) Canon Flint about the idea of me coming to live with her and her parents as they were planning a move from Stafford to a new area. The pressure on cot space must have been immense, as Canon Flint jumped at the suggestion, and hoped that my mother would collect me when she visited the following Sunday.

Sadly, a month later the hope had passed. My mother explained that fear and stigma continued to surround the risk of neighbours in Stafford discovering that she had had an illegitimate child. The colour of my skin, together with my mother's eventual plans to join my father in Nigeria, meant that I could not be passed off as a foster child despite her parents' support. It must have been a dreadful nightmare.

4 August 1949
Dear Canon Flint,

I think you will by this time have received a letter from our parish priest, Father Cregg. My mother has had a talk with him about the question of bringing Elizabeth to live with us, and he was very definitely against the idea, and promised to write to you to explain his point of view.

Unfortunately, I was unable to see either you or Father Murphy during my last visit to Coleshill, and so could not explain the position fully as I would have wished.

When I mentioned to you, some months ago, my intention of removing Elizabeth from the Home in the comparatively near future, I was under the impression that my father would be leaving Stafford, and that we could take her with us to a strange town where her appearance would cause less comment. This has not materialised, however, and it now seems that my family will be staying in Stafford indefinitely.

My mother thought that we might nevertheless bring Elizabeth here, and give people to understand that she was being looked after temporarily as a foster child, in response to the appeal for foster parents which has been read out in church recently. Father Cregg thinks, however, that this would be inadvisable, as people would not readily believe such a story.

I should explain that I am definitely engaged to marry Elizabeth's father, who has now returned to his home in Africa, as soon as he is in a better financial position. This may not be for a year or two, or longer, and in the meantime I really don't know what to do about Elizabeth.

As you know, only one or two people in Stafford know anything about the child. Even my two sisters know nothing, and my mother is very conscious that they should be kept in ignorance. Father Cregg seems quite convinced that, if Elizabeth comes here, no matter what story we tell, the truth will come out, with very unpleasant consequences for both my parents and my younger sisters. He points out, also, that whatever we say now will have to be contradicted later, when I get married and take Elizabeth away with me.

I would be very glad of your advice in this matter, as I now feel very undecided. I realise that I was a little hasty in writing to you on the subject in the first place, and that I shall be causing inconvenience by changing my mind now. Believe me, I am very sorry about this.

If Elizabeth's place is urgently wanted for another child, I will try to make some other arrangement, but I hope it will be possible for you to keep her for at least a few months longer. I have been thinking lately of trying to get work in some other town, with a view to having her with me, but there are a good many difficulties in the way.

Apologising once again for being such a trouble to you, and thanking you for all you have done for Elizabeth.

I am,

Yours sincerely,

Mary Furlong

PS I enclose £3 towards maintenance account. Will you

please send me a pass to see Elizabeth on Sunday, 14 August.

The powerful status and views of the Catholic clergy are clear. Goodness knows what my mother must have thought about Canon Flint's next piece of advice: to find a foster carer for me, who might be prepared to let her visit regularly. In the event, I stayed at the nursery until January 1951, during which time my mother gave her consent for me to have the diphtheria vaccine; I had bronchitis; and she was able to see me six times between April and December 1950. Then she received this update:

Dear Miss Furlong,

Owing to the great shortage of nursery accommodation, I have been obliged to transfer Elizabeth to Nazareth House, Rednal, Birmingham. You can rest assured that she will continue to receive the same care and attention which she received at Coleshill.

Visiting day at Rednal is the second Sunday for each month. I do not issue passes for this nursery.

I enclose directions from Birmingham.

Your maintenance contributions should be sent to me here as usual. With best wishes.

Yours sincerely,
Administrator WF/mf

So, my stay at Father Hudson's was to end as abruptly as it had begun.

Chapter 8:

To Nazareth House

Letter from Siobhán, the Origins social worker:

> . . . Then on 3 January 1951, you were transferred to
> Nazareth House, Rednal due to a shortage of nursery
> accommodation at Coleshill. Mary was advised of this change
> and given directions, so she could visit you there.

From the age of three and a half, I lived at Nazareth House
Catholic children's home and, to be honest, I can't even
remember the names of any of the nuns who looked after
me. It was on the Bristol Road in Birmingham, very close
to the huge green Lickey Hills Country Park, and one of
my fondest memories was walking with the other children
in a crocodile to the park, where we'd roll down the steep
grassy slopes.

Sunday was the day of the week I most dreaded, as it
meant having to go to Mass twice or, sometimes, even three
times. First, we would go to the children's Mass, followed in
the afternoon by the Benediction (the latter being the lesser
of the two evils). The worst type of Sunday would be if we
also had to attend the 11 o'clock Mass, as this was extremely
long and very boring. I took great pleasure in coming up
with various amusements to make the time go faster, or

at least make it more enjoyable while kneeling, sitting or standing in the pews. Making patterns with my rosary beads was always a favourite pastime, as I loved the feel of the shiny, coloured glass beads, and my imagination knew no bounds with the shapes that I could make.

Then, as she often could, my mum would visit on Sundays from 2 p.m. to 4 p.m. There wasn't even time to get excited, as the nuns were running the show and I was simply told: 'Elizabeth, your mum's here.'

I'd wait to meet her in the huge recreation hall where we had assemblies. It had gleaming, polished floors – everything was polished – I remember that because later on in my time there, I'd be doing the polishing. It had a stage with stairs leading up to it and, most probably, a cross (after all, it was a Catholic convent). I'd stand with a few other children who were not 'up for adoption'. I was aware that this made us different to the other larger group of children who were playing at the other end of the hall or outside. They'd be the focus of the adults who trooped in, and I later realised these people were coming to see if any of them were suitable for adoption.

I was never one of those children though – instead I was so proud of my mother, who was so beautiful and smartly dressed; what we'd call chic. She wore lipstick, which was always red, red, red, and kept her coat on so we could immediately leave together. I can't remember much else; I can't even remember if she wore high heels. But she would bend down to give me a hug; she was always affectionate but never loud in either emotions or physical contact.

Once together, we'd turn right out of the convent and usually go for a walk in Lickey Hills. We'd only be together a few hours, as she would travel to the convent and then home to her parents' house in Stafford in the same day. To a small child it seemed a long walk, but I bet now as an adult we'd get there in five minutes. That's my only memory of where we went – I do remember her buying me ice cream, so there must have been a van or cafe there, too.

However, her plan to marry my father wasn't to be. When she replied to my letter in 1994, my mother gave the impression that their relationship was a short-lived affair and he'd always planned to return to Nigeria: 'Shortly after our brief romance, he returned to Nigeria . . . We exchanged occasional letters, and I learned from one of these that he had married a lady of his own country.'

This doesn't tally with the correspondence of the time, talking about her engagement in her letter to Reverend Flint, and I just put it down to the fact that this period was so traumatic for her. It didn't turn out the way she wanted it to. Without the letters in the dossier, I would never have known that my parents' relationship had been longer and more affectionate than my mother had led me to believe.

From marrying my father to the plans to leave Stafford and bring me home and become a journalist, lots of her dreams just didn't come to fruition. Time after time, they would just fall apart. And I can't help thinking, *how did I come through all of this?* I think it was my mother's early presence and the kick-start I got from that. This was a family who was trying to keep everything together despite the obstacles in their way.

An image of her from that time has stayed with me; I still can't understand why it fascinated me so much. It was a freezing day and she was sneezing a lot and using a handkerchief. For one moment, though, a drip just hung from the tip of her nose and I wondered how long it would sit there. One more thing that always stayed with me was learning from her from an early age that 'she wanted to make a home for me'.

Chapter 9:
A Sense of Self

Nazareth House was opposite the huge Longbridge Austin car works factory in Rednal. One day, I could hear the lovely song 'Keep Right on to the End of the Road' (which I discovered is the anthem of Birmingham City Football Club) and lots of noise, which was very unusual. I remember asking one of the nuns what was happening and she replied, 'It's a strike.' 'What's a strike?' 'Oh, never you mind,' she replied. I think I got that from my mum – I was very, very inquisitive. When someone told me I couldn't know something, my first instinct was to go and find the answer.

This became a particular issue when it came to schooling. I wasn't allowed to start school with the other children as I was one of the youngest in the convent at the time, having been transferred to Nazareth House at a younger age than I should have been due to cot shortages at Father Hudson's Care.

I was really envious, seeing the other children troop into their classrooms. The nuns must have become very irritated with my constant nagging to be included. While waiting for this special day to arrive, one of the nuns took pity on me and took it upon herself to teach me to tell the time. There was a very large clock on the wall, and I was delighted when I managed to understand the difference between the fingers pointing to the hours, minutes and seconds and correctly tell her the time.

When I did finally start school – alongside children from the local area – the teacher was surprised to find that I could already read a bit. This was because one of my older friends realised that I loved to look at comics such as *The Beano* and used to help me to work out what some of the words meant. I regularly completed the spelling assessments, although repeatedly stumbled at the word 'knowledge'. A salutary lesson for me.

The rest of the time we used to be outside a lot and in all weathers, playing races, skipping games, hopscotch (my favourite), leapfrog, tag, conkers and marbles. Making daisy chains was another regular pastime, as was twirling buttercups under chins to see if friends wet the bed. I loved the countryside and, while scared of bulls, remember observing that rhubarb seemed to grow out of cow manure.

I can't remember much about the food, so it can't have been awful. One day I sneaked into the kitchens and, before being chased out, was suitably impressed by what looked like a huge potato-peeling machine going at great speed. I always thoroughly looked forward to the daily queuing up for doses of cod liver oil and malt extract, and we always had to brush our teeth using Gibbs Dentifrice, a pink paste contained in small tins. The more you rubbed the paste with your toothbrush, the more it frothed up, and I was often told off for using too much.

Very gradually, it became clear to me that my skin colour was not the same as all the other children's. When it was hot weather I always wanted to keep my cardigan on to hide my arms, which makes me laugh now as there was no logic to it, as my face, hands and legs would still have been showing. I didn't want people to see my skin colour or face the shame and stigma that surrounded it then.

Although I was generally a healthy child, I was referred to as a 'chesty child' – diagnosed as asthmatic when I was eleven – and suffered from quite severe bouts of eczema from a very early age. One day I ended up in the sick bay following my attempts to make my skin lighter than it was in order to look like all the other children. I had washed my face and arms at least ten times with red carbolic soap, and because of my sensitive skin, it had caused such a dreadful flare-up.

Thinking about it now, this really highlights how I felt different and 'other', and how I wanted to be the same as my friends. I bet there are lots of examples I could have used about being either subtly or more overtly identified as different because of the colour of my skin that I don't remember. I always give this example when I'm doing talks, because it really hits the audience. For a child to wash themselves ten times and hurt themselves really makes people understand what I'd experienced as a mixed-race child and how searing it was. Whether it's Black, brown or white people who have mixed-race children, this story really resonates with them and people latch onto it: 'My God, you actually wanted to change your external appearance.'

Many people of colour also tell me how pleased they are to hear a person like me, with status, openly talking about the stigma I experienced, because it's something quite deep. There are a lot of people who won't want to discuss it because being made to feel that way is so hurtful and embarrassing, and it feels like it should remain a secret. Maybe you've even grown up in a family who just don't want you to talk about it. Even if I can't remember all the times it happened – even if it was just a few times – it was enough that I wanted to change my skin colour.

I've always been open about it and, having grown up with all of that stigma and low self-esteem, now I'm at ease and content with who I am. However, if you don't come out of that experience well, it can knock you for six and affect your well-being, your career and your relationships. Now, I'd tell that child the same things I tell my daughter and granddaughter: that she should see the beauty of who she is, and that just because other people or society downgrade brown- and black-skinned individuals, that's their problem, not hers – and they're wrong for it.

I have other memories, too. Sitting cross-legged on the floor of the big hall, we were shown a film or slides by a missionary nun in a white habit of African children, and we were asked to pray for them. I remember some of the other children started pointing and laughing at me. It felt terrible because I was so embarrassed, mortified and angry, but there was nothing I could do about it. It was that sense of powerlessness that I couldn't just turn around and thump them – I had to suck it up, as they say.

Another time was when a nun, who I'd never viewed as particularly friendly, suddenly became very pally with me. I clearly remember when she crouched down and informed me that a new 'coloured' child was coming to join the convent. I'm not sure I even met the child, but I vividly remember being suspicious of this nun. A lot of people experience this (and it's not just to do with colour, it can be something like a disability), when people make assumptions about who you are because of the way you look. That patronising, 'Here's a nice friend for you,' when all you want to reply is, 'Up yours.'

One thing that's clear now was that the nuns had no idea how to deal with my hair. They soon gave up trying to use a normal comb, as I would be in floods of tears due to it being so painful. Instead, they would take a bunch of my hair and tightly tie a red ribbon around it. While it might have looked pretty, it made my scalp throb so much that, as soon as possible, I would loosen the wretched bow. I think they thought they were being helpful. But worse was to come when Nitty Nora, the nun who checked for head lice, tried to use a very fine-toothed comb on me with dire and painful results. Fortunately, unlike many of my friends, I never had an outbreak of nits or lice in my hair, so I was soon excused from this horrible procedure.

One of the clearest and most hurtful memories of the effects of being a Black child was when one nun overruled another who had chosen me to play Humpty Dumpty in a show that was being put on. She was of the opinion that Humpty Dumpty could not be Black. I sobbed so much that the decision was once more overturned, and I fell off that wall as the best and happiest Humpty Dumpty those nuns ever saw.

Chapter 10:

Faith and Hope

Religion played a huge role in life at Nazareth House, and I have vivid memories relating to the rituals and events that were part and parcel of a Catholic upbringing. The nuns played the most important part in my life at the convent, whereas priests were usually seen at the altar or from behind a grille in the confessional box. It was clear, though, that the nuns treated them like gods and were often at their beck and call.

Preparation for my first confession caused me confusion and anxiety when I was about seven years old, and had to tell the priest what sins I had committed. It didn't help that I didn't really understand what a sin was and that I felt under immense pressure to come up with a good one. The best that I could admit to was stealing somebody's comic. This wasn't very successful, as the priest gently pointed out that the comics belonged to all of the children in the house. Undeterred, I ploughed on, fabricating a story that I had fought with the child in order to read it. Satisfied with that, the priest gave me however many Hail Marys he thought necessary for my penance and I slipped away, chastened but feeling smug.

Looking back, one sin that I never confessed to was joining in with friends to make the life of one older nun

48

a great misery. After the lights were switched off, a check would be made to see that we had all settled down to sleep. There was one particular nun whose steps we always recognised, as she walked very slowly and with a stick. Shortly after entering the dormitory, a kid from the other end would start meowing and the nun would try to hobble over to find the culprit. Of course, the noise stopped before she reached the relevant bed and another one of us would start yapping like a dog down the other end. We were never caught but, fortunately for the nun, she was eventually relieved of these duties and the burden of dealing with such horrid children.

My first communion was an incredibly happy affair. There was huge excitement in the air, and I remember my lovely white dress and shoes, together with the most wonderful shiny white prayer book and new rosary beads. The only blip was when I chewed the host instead of swallowing it. One of the nuns pointed out to me that I had been eating God. I wasn't very upset, as even at that early age it didn't sense to me that God could be swallowed by all of the children. I loved the taste of the communion host, so much so that a group of us got into serious trouble by raiding a large box that contained the unblessed hosts. We were caught in the act when found with a fistful of them stuffed in our mouths.

The funniest and scariest game I got my friends to play with me took place when the priest gave out the Holy Communion, and the object was to see who could go up last to receive theirs. I usually won, as my trick was to make sure that I was seated at the end of the pew; I would wait until the priest thought that the last person had received their host and then, just as he turned back towards the altar, I would start running down the aisle towards him, timing it to perfection. Eventually, the priest complained to one of the nuns and I got a severe telling-off. It was worth it, though!

A nun used to give piano lessons to me and a few other children, and when we had played particularly well she would take us into Birmingham city centre for a Knicker-bocker Glory. These were sumptuous ice creams in what appeared to a small child to be very tall glasses and were eaten using a very long spoon. I always felt immense regret about never having further piano lessons after leaving the convent, but I have never forgotten some of the tunes the nun taught me, particularly Irish jigs, and today I still play them by ear. 'The Rakes of Mallow' had a huge impact and, later, when I was at my grandmother's house, it was one I always used to play.

The Irish influence of the Catholic nuns also came out in force when they taught Irish dancing to some of the children on a Saturday morning. I absolutely adored it and was over the moon when I was chosen to take part in competitions throughout the region, including Stoke-on-Trent. The excitement of wearing the green sparkly costumes and buckle shoes will always remain with me, together with the fast-paced and rhythmic music. To cap it all, I regularly won medals and was clearly the centre of attention, as it must have been an unusual sight to see a young brown-skinned girl in an Irish dance troupe. Maybe this is why I now love the Jamaican song 'Brown Girl in the Ring'. Quite often adults, mainly men, would press money into my hand, including half-crowns. To my horror, they were always taken from me by the nuns and I would never see the coins again. At times I thought life was unfair and often wondered what happened to the money.

One of the things to make up for some of the downsides of life at Nazareth House were regular holidays, when we would swap our accommodation with children from a different convent. My favourite trip was to Nazareth House in Crosby, near Liverpool, as it was very close to the seaside. We would travel by coach and although I would often suffer from travel sickness, this was soon forgotten when I saw the sea. The sight of the blue water never failed to thrill me, and it still does.

Another trip that has always remained with me was the time we went to Evesham in Worcestershire and saw fruit orchards for the very first time – I particularly remember the apple trees. It may have been on this visit that we were taken to see the shrine to Our Lady of Evesham, where I met a monk and was chastised by one of the nuns for daring to ask what he wore under his brown habit. It wasn't the first time I had made such a mistake – I also got into hot water for asking whether nuns had any hair under their veils, or were they bald.

Some of my favourite times in Birmingham were visits from the Bournville Cadbury's chocolate factory staff, who would show us films such as *Laurel and Hardy* – which I really adored – and bring along chocolate for us. My favourite was the very small bar wrapped in purple paper, and the memory of opening and eating them still reminds me of Roald Dahl's book *Charlie and the Chocolate Factory*.

In June 1953, we were all made to watch the whole of the coronation of Queen Elizabeth II in black and white on a television. I would have been nearly six years of age and all I can recall is seeing lots of ladies walking around wearing white gowns. Also, the Queen looking very tiny to have such a large crown on her head, and the programme going on, and on, and on. Around the same time, there was great rejoicing at the news that the New Zealander

Edmund Hillary and the Nepalese Sherpa Tenzing Norgay had conquered Mount Everest on 29 May.

What took place at Christmas each year should easily come to mind, but for whatever reason, that's not the case. There was only one year that stands out. We were all in the large recreation hall, and when our names were called we went up to the nun at the Christmas tree to receive a present. Mine was some sort of doll. It was a huge disappointment and made me cry – which makes me think that our Christmas presents were usually of a much higher standard.

Meanwhile, my mother visited as often as she could, every month and sometimes more. The dossier from Father Hudson's Care meticulously listed her payments for my care and the dates she visited, which became more frequent as the years went by.

Chapter 11:

Future Foundations

One Sunday, the thought of attending so many religious services was just too much for me, so I decided to hide under my bed while all the other children went off to the chapel. My name was being called out, but I didn't move and kept as quiet as possible. Unfortunately, unaware that I was allergic to house dust, I suddenly started to have a violent sneezing attack. I was dragged out and marched off to Mass and received no sympathy (or handkerchief, for that matter, for my running eyes and nose).

My allergy meant that sweeping up dust made me feel very ill, but one nun was insistent that I should carry on despite my discomfort. Fortunately, another sister could see my distress and took me to see the Mother Superior, who agreed that I could be excused from this household chore. The alternative was great fun, as dusters were wrapped around my shoes to help me shine newly waxed corridor floors.

I regularly visited the sick bay for eczema treatments to see the 'white nun', so-called because she wore a white habit rather than a black one. The areas most affected were my elbow creases and, in those days, the treatment consisted of covering the red, itchy and painful skin with coal tar paste, followed by bandaging. Removing the bandages caused me great anxiety, as they would be stuck to the dry skin and the procedure could hurt a great deal.

I was so impressed with the way the 'white nun' always managed to distract me by using words that (at this tender age) seemed to be very rude, and not what you would expect to hear from such a holy person. Saying the word 'bottom' – it always made me laugh – just at the moment she took the bandages off never failed to work. Then came the best part of the procedure, when the new dressing was applied. It was so cool and soothing, making me forget all the previous discomfort.

The main thing was that she didn't cause me any pain; I think children in particular love that. I wasn't a sick-sick child, but I can imagine that for children with serious disabilities or chronic conditions that placed them in the hands of health personnel frequently, it's important that those people are good-humoured and funny. Anything humorous that an adult does that you don't expect is joyous; I'm pretty sure that's why that nun left such an imprint on me.

I'm never entirely sure when I decided I wanted to become a nurse, but I was fascinated by what they did. I used to feign injury so I could go and get bandages in the sick bay. Hot foments were applied to my chest when I was suffering breathlessness and coughing fits, and I'd also use a ceramic inhaler called Dr Nelson's Inhaler, filled with a brown tincture, to help my breathing. Just before I had my tonsils out, I can recall being on a trolley and smelling various vapours before being anaesthetised – the promise being kept that I would be able to eat loads of ice cream and jelly afterwards, which made the subsequent sore throat more bearable. Later on, at sixth form, when my teachers were encouraging me to go to university, I was dead set on nursing, so it must have been there all along.

A sadder memory I have is the first time I experienced the death of another child in the home, and the vague recollection that she had succumbed to leukaemia. It's a stark memory, of us all lined up the path as the funeral car carrying the girl's coffin drove out of the convent grounds. I remember feeling incredibly sad and scared. And that's when I first learned about this word, leukaemia; I must have been such a curious kid, because I definitely knew it was cancer. It could have been me being nosey, listening into conversations around me – as children you learn an awful lot from adults when they don't realise that you can hear what they're talking about.

Despite the inspiration of this kind nurse, the very worst memories I have are how the nuns dealt with children like me who wet the bed. First, we had to stand on a chair, then the urine-soaked bed sheet would be draped over our heads and we would have to lift our arms out and stand very still. If they should start to drop one iota, we would be rapped with a ruler. I knew even then that this was not something that the Catholic nuns should be doing. I frequently wet the bed and the trauma of this punishment remains stark.

As a health visitor, you often meet families whose children wet the bed, and there is now a real emphasis on not punishing children, because they're not doing it deliberately; I have such empathy for them. For one thing, you can make it worse by increasing children's sense of shame and anxiety. I remember that feeling of waking up and thinking, *oh no, it's happened again.*

It was such a cruel treatment and I often wonder, were they trained to do this? Nobody would have explored the psychology or physiology of it. Reading a 2005 memoir by another Nazareth House child, Judith Kelly, who lived in Essex in the early 1950s, she describes the punishment of a child called Janet who had wet her bed.[1] Like me, she had to remain in the dormitory and stand with the wet sheet over her head. I can imagine that the nuns would have learned the punishments from each other.

Since then, there have been some horrendous accounts of the treatment of children. As part of the 2019 Scottish Child Abuse Inquiry, the Nazareth Houses in Aberdeen, Glasgow, Midlothian and Ayrshire were censured by the chairlady, who said: 'The Nazareth Houses in Scotland were, for many children, places of fear, hostility and confusion, places where children were physically abused and emotionally degraded with impunity. There was sexual abuse of children which, in some instances, reached levels of the utmost depravity. Children in need of kind, warm, loving care and comfort did not find it. Children were deprived of compassion, dignity, care and comfort.'[2] Barry Adams was six years old in December 1959 when he arrived at the same Nazareth House I had left three years earlier. In his traumatic 2004 memoir, *Pater Noster*, he refers to it as 'Nazi House'.[3]

Most damning of all was my later discovery that Canon Flint, who had been so supportive to my mother and grandparents, was instrumental in the child migration scheme.[4] This programme was responsible for sending 130,000 children to Britain's former colonies such as Australia and Canada between the 1920s and the 1970s, where many suffered sexual, physical and emotional abuse. A report by the Independent Inquiry into Child Sexual Abuse revealed that 39 of 132 children were selected from Nazareth House between 1947 and 1956 for the scheme, and that Father Hudson's Care should have done more to protect the children by following up on post-migration monitoring.[5] The report also stated that Canon Flint, who died in 1982, signed migration forms as both the sponsoring organisation and a child's guardian, which raises questions around a conflict of interest, 'especially when that person appeared to be a powerful advocate for child migration'.

One boy, Raymond Brand, was admitted to Coleshill at the age of five months in May 1948, arriving just after me. When his mother could no longer afford his care, Father Hudson's Care suggested he should be put up for adoption, but instead he was sent to Western Australia on RMS *Oronsay* in 1953, aged five. There, he was beaten and abused in a number of orphanages and wasn't reunited with his stepbrothers until 1994. His devastating story is now housed in the Australian National Maritime Museum in Sydney. [6] In the context of these stories, I was incredibly lucky in my experience of Nazareth House, as my close relationship with my mother would have protected me.

In 2020, another child, Ann Sweeney, who lived locally and attended the St Brigid's Annexe school at Nazareth House, contacted me saying she'd heard about me being on the BBC radio show *Desert Island Discs*, talking about the Lickey Hills. Ann sent me this picture, on the following page, of us in a class photo aged about seven or eight with a nun standing at either side of the group, and I'm the only Black kid in it.

Ann wasn't sure why I had made such an impression on her but, as she was an extremely quiet, shy child, she thought it could be because I was talkative. She recalls sitting next to me and that I was kind to her. Ann also remembers asking her parents why my skin was brown. They explained that everybody is different in some way, for example some people are tall while others are short. She told me that she'd been upset when I left Nazareth House suddenly in 1956; at aged nine, my mother was finally in a position to bring me home.

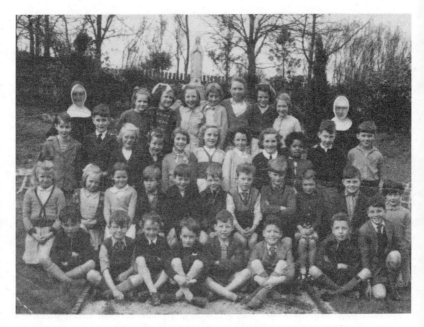

Me at school while at Nazareth House.

On 14 August 1956, my mother wrote her final letter to Nazareth House:

Dear Canon Flint,

As mentioned in my last letter, we have got a house, and my husband and I are both very anxious that Elizabeth should come home as soon as possible. I shall be leaving my job on August 31st, and by that time Elizabeth's room should be furnished and everything ready for her. I cannot adequately express my gratitude to you and the sisters for your care of Elizabeth during the past nine years but, as you know, it has always been my wish to have her with me as soon as circumstances permitted.

I hope, therefore, that it will be quite convenient for me to call for her on Sunday, September 2nd.

The clearest memory I have of this momentous day was the journey to Wolverhampton with my mother to start this new life with her and her new husband. We took a bus from Birmingham and were seated on the lower deck at the back near the stairs to the upper deck. I was absolutely distraught at leaving my friends and the convent – the only home I had ever known – and started to sob uncontrollably. The conductor was clearly concerned and asked my mother why I was so upset.

She tried to explain, but I think it must have been extremely embarrassing for her, and also quite painful, in view of all the obstacles she had overcome in her efforts to provide a home for me at last. Little did either of us know that over the next twenty months, I would be shedding many, many more tears.

Chapter 12:

Mum and Ken

Letter from Siobhán, the Origins social worker, 14 September 2011:

In August 1953, Mary wrote to advise us she had got married and was now Mary Hart (living in Wolverhampton) and that her husband would take responsibility for making payments towards your keep. They applied for a council house with a view to being able to have you come to live with them. By August 1956, Mary had a house in Low Hill, Wolverhampton. She then finished her job on 31 August and, on 2 September 1956, had you home from Nazareth House, after arranging for your discharge. So that completes the information we have about your background.

In September 1956, a couple of months after my ninth birthday, I moved to Wolverhampton to finally live with my mother and her husband, Ken. Stepping into my new home for the first time, I was struck by the fact that there were no photos or flowers on the mantelpiece. Maybe this vision of a typical family home had come from children's books, such as the Janet and John series, which I'd read so avidly in the convent; I was incredibly disappointed and felt bitterly let down. It was not the most auspicious start.

Aged thirty-one, Ken was originally from Bolton and had come from a poor working-class family. Ken's father, John Hart, had been a mill hand and a gambler, and his mother struggled to make ends meet. My sister Marion recalled Ken telling her his dad had picked up his wages at the end of the week and gambled the lot on a horse. He lost it and, of course, in those days there was no social security. His mum had to feed them and send them to school every day with something to eat and, basically, neighbours helped each other out. His mother baked bread and that's how she got by.

Having found work as a builder's labourer in Bolton, Ken had married and had a son called Kenny, who was nine months younger than me, but it had ended in a bitter divorce. Marion told me it had been a terrible trauma for him because he'd been so besotted with his first wife.

Ken joined the Royal Air Force and was posted to Gibraltar for two years before being transferred to a base in Stafford. There, in 1952, he met my mother at a firemen's ball in the town. I remember seeing a photograph of him looking very smart in his air force uniform – he must have cut a dashing figure.

They were married at the Wolverhampton Register Office on 8 August 1953, and my grandfather was the only member of her family to attend (as a witness to the ceremony, his signature is included in the register book). My younger brother Mick was born three months later, but the marriage was hampered by problems from the start. My mother's account to me in 1994 explains why:

My marriage caused a rift with my parents, which never really healed. My husband had divorced his first wife after a brief and disastrous marriage. This meant that the Catholic Church

*would not recognise his marriage to me, and in my parents'
eyes I was proposing to live in sin, cut off from any hope of
salvation. I could understand their attitude, knowing what the
Catholic doctrine was, but I had had enough of living under
a cloud of disapproval and in an atmosphere of secrecy. My
husband had been offered a job in Wolverhampton on leaving
the Air Force, and we went into lodgings there until we were
allotted a council house.*

*As we had agreed at the time of our engagement, you
came to live with us as soon as we had accommodation, as did
the son of my husband's first marriage. By that time, we had
a baby son, and another child was on the way.*

As a result of marrying a divorced man, who was also a
Protestant, my mother was barred from receiving Holy
Communion. My brother and sister recall that every Sunday
without fail, the family still went to Mass. When Holy Communion was given, everyone got out of his or her pew; row
after row went up, but Mum had to stay alone in her seat.

As well as Mick, Frank was born in 1957, eight months
after I moved to Wolverhampton (my younger sisters Marion
and Pam were born later, in 1961 and 1962). Kenny was also
living with us (according to my brother Frank, Ken had
wanted custody of his son partly out of revenge on his first
wife). It must have been quite cramped with four children
and two adults, and the pram at the bottom of the stairs.
Fortunately, all of us children got on well.

Frank's arrival made me extremely happy, as he was such
a gorgeous plump and cheerful blue-eyed little boy. I loved
playing with him, and we developed a special bond. Mick
was six years younger than me and was a gentle and quiet
boy who loved playing football. I also got on well with

Kenny. At some point he left Wolverhampton, but I don't know when or the details, except that he had returned to his own mother when her circumstances improved.

Our house was on a council estate in Low Hill and was the first major housing development of its kind in Wolverhampton. By 1927, it consisted of more than 2,000 new council houses and was one of the largest housing estates in Britain at the time. But, over the years, it acquired an increasingly bad reputation and, by the time my family had moved in, there was a lot of poverty.

Ours was the second along a terrace of four houses, and to get to our back door we had to walk round the side of the neighbour's house and across their backyard. It was small even by today's standards. Downstairs there was a tiny hallway. The living room had a lino floor and was the biggest room, heated by a coal fire. There was no heating anywhere else in the house. The black and white television set stood in the corner of the living room; there was a sofa and Ken's armchair.

A pantry off the living room featured a concrete slab to keep the milk and butter cool. Mum kept everything in there: food, ironing basket, coats and shoes. There was no fridge while I lived there; they didn't buy one until the 1970s. A door next to the pantry led into the kitchen, with a cooker and a clothes rack above, a table and a sink unit under the window. Before she finally got a washing machine, I remember Mum washing the clothes by hand and putting them through a wringer to remove as much water as possible before hanging them on the rack or outside on the washing line.

Off the kitchen was the coalhouse, about the same size as the pantry. The bathroom was also off the kitchen and, as well as a bath, there was a big green gas boiler with a tap above. We filled it up to heat the water and had to ladle the water into the bath. This was a slow and colossal task, so it's not surprising that having a bath was only a weekly event. The back door led from the kitchen out to the yard, which had a shed where Ken kept his tools and ladders. The back garden was surrounded by hedges and was turfed with a central path. It was always overgrown, as neither Mum nor Ken had the time or energy for gardening.

The presence of large Alsatian dogs roaming around the neighbourhood seemed to be the order of the day. I was petrified of the constant barking, as well as of their black bushy eyebrows. I was always fearful of going outside the kitchen door, whether to go round the neighbour's house to reach the street or just to get to the outside toilet – speed was essential. The toilet was freezing cold in the winter, and there were only squares of newspaper hanging from a nail, instead of toilet paper.

There were three bedrooms: Mum and Ken had the largest one at the front and the other two, at the back of the house, were very small; I slept in one of them. It could be freezing at times and I absolutely hated being cold, especially as it brought on my wheezing attacks. My asthma had not yet been diagnosed, but I was always 'chesty'. A freezing outdoor toilet and a cold bedroom would not have helped, nor the fact that Mum and Ken were heavy smokers. To add to my woes, pea-souper fogs were still a frequent occurrence in this industrial area of the West Midlands.

Frank was also affected: 'No wonder you and I had asthma, as it was a smoky place due to the coal fire and Mum and Dad always smoking. There were so many factories in the Low Hill area that had chimneys belching smoke out all the time. There was the Goodyear Tyre factory, which caused a stink around the place, and there was also a smelting furnace works.' The Clean Air Act was passed in 1956, but it would take many years before pollution-triggered fogs became a rare event.

After Ken left the RAF, he had a number of jobs before settling down to long-distance lorry driving, but he was constantly moving from one haulage firm to another. Lack of money meant my mother had to get a job, too. It was unusual for women to work when they were married, but Mum took office jobs: first at the Electric Construction Company and then at Goodyear, both of which dominated the landscape. It wasn't equal pay in those days, so Mum took home half the amount a man would have earned doing the same job then had to give half of that to the childminder over the road.

Years later, Mum told me how pleased she was to be asked to use her linguistic skills at work, but I was furious that it was never appropriately recompensed. She worked in the traffic office at Goodyear, although it was quite a menial clerk's job. The managers found out that she could speak German and Italian, so when the foreign drivers came in and they couldn't understand them, they used to call Mum down from the traffic office to do the interpreting. Later, Mum discovered that she could have been paid a lot more for this work, but it never happened.

That money would really have come in handy, as poverty was a constant and grinding reality. She always had a look of worry about money and, coming from Nazareth House, I didn't expect to be given pocket money and knew not to ask for things. Day-to-day shopping had to be put on a tab until Friday, when she received her wages and could settle all the bills, while clothes were bought via a catalogue and the TV had a meter for money. I remember people coming to the door to collect what was owed. It makes me wonder how the expenses of daily living were divided up between her and Ken. My brother Frank felt that Ken kept at least half of his wages to spend down at the pub.

Mum never drank but, as with many of their generation, they both smoked heavily. Cigarettes seemed to offer one way of helping her to deal with stress. Once, when she was upset over something, my brother Mick, who was a lovely-natured little boy and very sensitive, said: 'Mum, sit down, read book, have moke [a smoke].' I also loved reading, and there would be times when both my mother and I were curled up with books in the living room, which Ken would resent.

It always seemed a terrible shame that Mum was unable to use her academic abilities. I was very angry about this and I went through a period when I really couldn't understand why she wasn't more assertive and seemed to be in this subservient role to Ken. She was obviously so much brighter than that, and as a young child it didn't make any sense to me. This frustration stopped me looking up to her slightly, and I wanted to know the answer why – I always do. But as a child you don't always know the background of things.

When Ken was home – he'd often be away driving or at the pub – he loved television and would be the one to comment on the programmes, deciding what we'd watch; there weren't many channels to choose from. Saturday afternoon seemed to be dominated by wrestling on ITV – a sport I came to hate with a vengeance. It was utterly mindless, watching huge men in skimpy outfits throwing each other around the ring and then leaping on top of their opponents with a deadening thud. But we'd all watch *Sunday Night at the London Palladium* together (everyone did then) and he'd be cracking jokes. You could see why my mother found Ken attractive. He had a good sense of humour – and in that early stage when he drank, he was very funny, happy and good to be around. He knew he was good-looking and he had a shock of black hair, which he'd Brylcreem, and a little moustache. He looked after his appearance.

Lunch was bread and dripping every day, and one of my responsibilities was to go to the local infant welfare clinic to exchange coupons for tins of National Dried Milk for Frank and orange juice in glass bottles. The only other major errand I can vaguely remember involved walking some distance wheeling a trolley to collect coal.

The street was my playground, and people were generally friendly. In good weather I can recall sitting down on the pavement and just watching the world go by. My favourite pastime was going to St Christopher's Penny Bike Park in Fifth Avenue to learn road safety. Everything was child-sized and roads were laid out with traffic lights and zebra crossings. It was within easy walking distance and a very cheap way to ride a bike. I spent hours there and it was huge fun.

Records show that my first day at school was Monday, 3 September 1956 – just one day after leaving Nazareth House. I was enrolled at St Mary's Roman Catholic Junior School. I have hardly any memories of my time at this school, apart from joining a library and the fact that there was no uniform. Instead, I always wore the same yellow dress, day in and day out, all week. It was such a relief when it was washed at the weekend, so much so that I loved Mondays and Tuesdays, as the dress would always feel fresh and clean.

I experienced two severe 'bronchial' episodes at that time. The first was when my auntie Pat finally came to meet me for the first time when I was ill and also hallucinating. She later recalled: 'It was in 1956 and I was nineteen. My mum told me about you on the train going to see you, and you were in bed so I didn't really have a conversation with you because you were very chesty. I gathered from the conversation that we did have that you thought I was your teacher.'

The second episode, around 1956 or 1957, brought home to me how poor we really were. Prescription charges had been introduced for everyone in 1952 at a shilling per pre-scription, and then in 1956 it was increased to two shillings per item; it would seem there were no exemptions for me as a child.[1] The local doctor was examining me in the front room and asked my mum if she had obtained some medicine he'd recommended for me during his previous visit. While she was trying to explain there wasn't enough money to pay for it, he exploded in anger, giving her some money and telling her to go to the chemist immediately. It was a shocking moment, and I will never ever forget feeling so ashamed and embarrassed for my mother.

Chapter 13:
Dark Days

Lentil soup day was definitely one I used to fear. Although it was a tasty dish, it was cooked in the dreaded pressure cooker, which could explode when the lid blew off. The soup would splatter all over the kitchen ceiling, so I was always scared of hearing the hissing noise and seeing the black button rising from the top of the pressure cooker lid.

I can see my mum standing in the kitchen over the soup with a book in her hand. She could switch off even when we were all in the living room and Ken was at home; if he was there, you knew he was there, acting like the 'man of the house'. Mum would just be quiet but cheerful in his presence; she had the better of him and wasn't a doormat, but she was also good at keeping the peace. She made sure the children didn't annoy him by being too noisy and kept a careful balancing act. She was very warm but she was also very introverted in terms of her book reading; I didn't understand it then, but she could juggle living in a small council house while cooking, shopping and working, as long as she had her books.

However, life started slowly to become more miserable as Ken began to treat me differently from his own children. The first example etched in my mind was one hot day when he bought everybody ice creams except me. I sat on the pavement outside and just cried. It appeared that he enjoyed being awkward with me and asking the impossible; it felt that nothing I did would ever be right. Once, I was in the kitchen doing the washing-up and trying to dry some glasses, without much success as the tea towel was damp. He kept asking me to dry them again and again, and when I pointed out the problem with the tea towel, he tore it from my hand and hit me with it.

Unknown to me, it would seem that Ken couldn't cope with the taunts at work about my presence in the home. According to Pat, 'You were having trouble when Ken was having remarks made to him at work – from what I could gather – that you were Black, and what was he letting his wife do. He wasn't the sort of bloke who could take that sort of thing.' At that time in Wolverhampton – before the increase of Caribbean emigration at the end of the 1950s and beginning of the 1960s – I was still unusual.

I started to become scared of him, as he began to lash out and slap me for no good reason, often when my mum wasn't around. He had severe mood swings, which were always due to drink. I used to dread his return to the house, stinking of beer and smoke, and quickly learned to gauge his state of drunkenness. The least fearful was when he was slightly tipsy, grinning and telling jokes. In the past, this would have heralded a time of laughter with all the family but, later, I would be on guard as his mood could change at any moment. The darker stage began when he became argumentative and angry, and my mum and I would both be in the firing line.

Frank remembers that Ken 'could be complimentary or cruel. Once he had had a bit to drink, he would be happy and hug us all. When he'd had too much, his character would change and he could be a verbal bully and unpredictable. He was like a firework. The worst times were when he was so broke that he couldn't afford to smoke or go down to the pub to drink. I learned to fight very quickly and was a bit of a lad, trespassing over the gasworks. Mick was a real gentleman, but his aggression was channelled into his football and athletics.'

One day it must have all got too much for Mum, as she left the house, pushing Frank in his pram, with me and Mick alongside. We walked and walked, to a police station if my memory serves me right, but I can't remember what happened next. We obviously returned home, and it was the only time it happened. Frank remembers, when he was about eight, being very scared one Sunday afternoon and running to a neighbour's house for help. Ken was drunk and had lost his temper with Mum and started dragging her by her hair.

Frank told me that Ken used to keep a belt with his overalls on a hook on the coalhouse door, and would use it on Micky, Kenny and him. In contrast, Marion only remembers him shouting at her or Pam, but never striking them. She never saw him ever use any violence against Mum, but when asked about this, Mum replied that when the children were a lot younger, he did once raise his hand to her. My mum picked up a broom and threatened him with it, warning him that if he ever laid a hand on her, he would never see her again. Ken backed off, not saying a word, and never tried that again.

My mother's account of what led to my grandparents taking me in was at odds with what I remembered: 'As the next few years went by, I became worried about your future. You were obviously highly intelligent, and in our difficult financial circumstances, with other children competing for the available money and attention, it seemed unlikely that we could give you the sort of start in life that you deserved and needed. My parents had moved to Wallasey, a pleasant residential district of the Merseyside area where they had grown up. Their children were on their own feet, as one of my sisters had entered a convent and the other had qualified as an accountant. They kindly offered to have you to live with them until you were sixteen, as Wallasey could offer a more middle-class background and better educational opportunities.'

My recollection was of a more brutal denouement that led to me being rescued by my grandparents and is forever etched in my memory. The incident that was apparently the last straw took place one night after Ken had come home from the pub. I was by this time fast asleep upstairs. Mum told him that I'd kicked Mick earlier in the day, although for the life of me I cannot remember why I'd lashed out at my younger brother in this way. Perhaps poor Mick was on the receiving end of my pent-up frustrations. Whatever the reason, Ken was so angry that he came upstairs to wake me up and then dragged me down the stairs to the front room. I was absolutely terrified. He struck me so hard that I fell across the room and hit my eyebrow on the edge of the metal hearth. I don't think he deliberately aimed to injure me – he just slapped me so hard I went flying across this small room. It bled profusely and, to this day, it still hurts if I touch the spot above my left eye.

This incident must have been the breaking point for my poor mother, who probably also felt enormous guilt at what had happened. She contacted my grandparents and sought their help, as this was a step too far. It was the worst incident of physical abuse I'd had from my stepfather, and they immediately came and rescued me. I didn't know it then, but my auntie Pat later told me that my grandmother had never liked Ken and thought that he'd treated me very unfairly.

It's probably one of the factors why I've turned out not to be too screwed up by things: my grandparents were very caring and even when my mother let them down by getting pregnant out of wedlock a second time, with Ken, they were still very supportive and came to my rescue when she and I needed them. A lot of families would have washed their hands of the whole situation. Some mothers would have been too scared to contact their parents, but I think it was desperation on my mother's part; she had no friends or close relatives she could call on (her brother was away at sea and her sisters were much younger). It also really underlines the bond she had with her parents, that she could still turn to them.

I wasn't exactly certain of the date when my rescue took place, but with the help of Wolverhampton Archives and Local Studies records and my sister Marion remembering the name of my school, I discovered that St Mary's Roman Catholic Junior School's admission had my last attendance noted on 9 May 1958; I would transfer to St Alban's Roman Catholic Junior School in Wallasey. Granddad came to collect me from Wolverhampton, and while sad to leave my mum and brothers, I was overjoyed to leave a house that held so many awful memories.

Chapter 14:

Rescued by My Grandparents

So two months short of my eleventh birthday in May 1958, I started a new phase of my life. I have absolutely no recollection of leaving Wolverhampton with my grandfather and travelling to Wallasey; even now, I don't really understand why this momentous journey has been obliterated from my memory.

Located on the other side of the River Mersey from Liverpool, Wallasey was often referred to as a dormitory town for commuters who would drive through the Mersey tunnel or go by ferry. I will never forget the contrast of my new home to the one in Low Hill. A semi-detached house located on Mill Lane in the Liscard area, it seemed huge to me.

I was now going to live with my grandfather, grandmother and Auntie Pat – my mother's youngest sister, who was only ten years older than me. Pat told me about my arrival: 'You were very quiet. I think you were rather flabbergasted. The thing I remember the most was that Mum nearly cried when she unpacked your suitcase because there was so little in it, and what there was wasn't fantastic. She took you out to Marks & Spencer one Saturday and kitted you out with new underwear.'

Pat came with us on that shopping expedition, and it was one that I would never, ever forget. It was the first time that

I remembered ever having been taken shopping for clothes. The store appeared immense and very bright, and there were so many beautiful clothes hung on see-through plastic hangers. Pants and vests were purchased alongside crisp white shirts, white socks, grey skirts, cardigans and black shoes for my new school uniform. My poor brain just could not take it all in.

I was admitted to St Alban's Roman Catholic Junior School for the few remaining months of the summer term, so it's not surprising that I have virtually no recollection of my time there. I can just about picture the iron railings surrounding the small playground and also attending Mass at the church next door.

I was thrilled to discover that my grandmother was exactly how I'd imagined she should look. Short and plump, with the most wonderful smile and great sense of humour, she always dressed in bright colours. When preparing to go out, I'd watch how she'd position her hat with a large and dangerous pin, worrying whether she would pierce her head with it.

My new home also left me in wonder. I remember that the gate opened up to a short path that led through a small garden up to a red front door with a large brass handle. Later on, it would be my duty to make sure this handle always shone brightly, a task that I thoroughly enjoyed. I loved the smell of the liquid Brasso, pouring some onto a cloth, rubbing it on, seeing it go white and then giving it a good old polish. Watching the drab handle become a bright, shiny gold colour gave me enormous satisfaction.

There was a small hall containing an umbrella stand, a telephone on a tiny table and a place to hang coats. On the wall, in a prominent position, was a large colour photograph

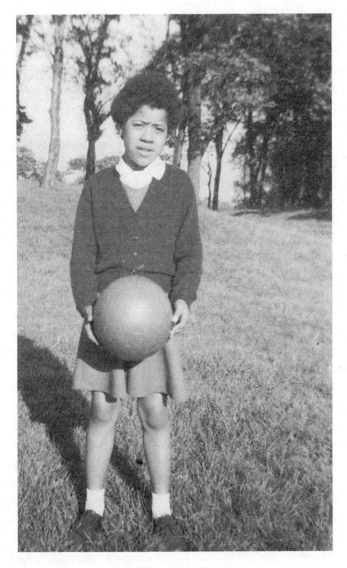

Me, aged eleven, in Wallasey.

of my grandfather sat astride a camel, posing in front of the pyramids, taken in Egypt during the First World War.

Carpeted stairs led up to a landing, where there was a bathroom and four bedrooms; one of which would be mine. Downstairs there was a front room, a dining room and a large kitchen. The latter was divided up into three sections. There was a pantry adjacent to a very cosy area heated by a coal fire and with a large Formica table and chairs where we generally ate. The radio was usually on, and I could look across to the cooking and washing-up area and chat to my grandmother as she prepared the food. A door led outside from here to an additional toilet, a bicycle shed and a large back garden. The dining room was at the back of the house and was only used for special occasions. We even had a gorgeous little terrier, Whisky.

I would spend most of my time with my grandmother, and she always appeared to be smiling and laughing. Religion was very important to her and she was incredibly respectful towards the local priests, attending Mass regularly. I loved her cooking, in particular her soda bread, lemon meringues and currant buns. Baking the latter was always a treat. A small amount of mixture was always left for me to spoon out into a special bun case and, once baked, I was able to eat it straightaway. It was the first time I had ever been asked to help in a kitchen and we would have great chats together.

The school was also in Mill Lane and just ten minutes' walk away, so I was able to come home for lunch. This was always very enjoyable, not only for my gran's lovely cooking, but also because we could listen to the radio while we ate – music and singing were a balm to me. It started when watching a film about the life of the waltz king Johann Strauss the Younger at school, when I fell in love with the

'Blue Danube' waltz. After that, I wanted to hear more music by Strauss, so I would pore over the *Radio Times* to see when any of his work was being played.

My grandmother was happy for me to twiddle with the radio buttons and tune into a concert. They seemed quietly bemused by my love for music. There was always a thrill when discovering new works such as the 'Tritsch-Tratsch' and 'Thunder and Lightning' polkas – and I quickly discovered other music by Schubert, Mozart, Beethoven and Dvořák. Later on, at secondary school, when striding into a morning assembly one day, I was delighted to recognise that it was to the resounding rhythm of Franz Schubert's 'Marche Militaire'.

The radio was a great source of entertainment. Saturday morning, for example, meant it was time for *Children's Favourites* with Uncle Mac. Many years later, I would introduce my daughter to some of the songs heard regularly on this show, such as 'Nelly the Elephant' and 'There's a Hole in the Bucket'. The humour of Ken Horne and his team on the brilliant comedy series *Beyond Our Ken* suited me down to the ground, although most of the double entendres went over my head. In contrast, I couldn't stand it when Billy Cotton bellowed out 'Wakey, Wakey!' as it also heralded the start of his *Band Show* programme that, to my mind, was never very entertaining. I preferred listening to comedy and a wide range of most types of music, a habit that has lasted to this day – I was never to be a Radio 4 listener.

As the months went on, my grandfather and I developed a close and warm friendship. To begin with he seemed rather a stern figure to me, quite tall and very engrossed in his newspaper and doing the crossword, so I was in awe of him. Plus, I hadn't been around any positive male role models. I was quite taken with how smartly he dressed and that he always wore a hat at a rakish angle. But it didn't take me long to realise that he had a wonderful sense of humour – he would tell me so many jokes, which lay the foundations of our friendship. I was also very, very curious and listened closely to what he said, which encouraged him to tell me stories, as I was a captive audience.

On our walks together, he discovered that I was interested in history and would talk to me about Ireland. He was pleased that I loved to listen to Irish music and he would explain to me the meaning of some of the songs. One was 'The Wearing of the Green', concerning the banning of the shamrock. The opening verse is:

> *Oh, Paddy dear, did you hear the news that's going 'round?*
> *The shamrock is forbid by law to grow on Irish ground*
> *Saint Patrick's Day no more to keep, his colour can't be seen.*
> *For there's a bloody law again' the Wearing of the Green.*

The arrival of a small parcel of shamrock from Ireland was an annual event, and my gran would pray fervently that it would come in time for St Patrick's Day on 17 March. We would all have a bunch pinned to our coats.

It won't come as a surprise, therefore, that Sunday was a very busy day, first going to Mass, followed by a classic Irish fry-up for breakfast. This was my introduction to black pudding, which I loved so much in those days. The wonderful smell of sizzling bacon, fried eggs, tomatoes and toast meant we would be soon called to sit at the kitchen table. Sunday lunch was always a succulent roast joint accompanied by vegetables, roast potatoes and gravy. If I was in luck, the most delicious lemon meringue pie would then follow. It is clear from the few photos of me from this period that I quickly put on a bit of a weight.

As usual, the radio would be on and we would listen to *Two-Way Family Favourites*. I was fascinated by the letters that were read out from families who wanted a special request for a relative in the armed forces (usually based in Cyprus or Germany). This was when I first came across the beautiful voice of African-American singer Paul Robeson, as his rendition of 'Ol' Man River' was frequently played. (Paul Robeson was a person who had a huge impact on me later in life; the US government stripped him of his passport after he refused to sign a 'loyalty oath', a move that was widely seen as punishment for his vocal civil rights support and refusal to denounce the Soviet Union. He's one of my heroes now.)

The front room was where I found other sources of entertainment that would keep me occupied for hours. The most exciting discovery was the pianola, which included a mechanism for inserting pianola rolls punched with perforations. A huge number of these rolls were stored inside the piano stool, and it was a journey of discovery picking one out at random and slotting it into place. I can see myself now, just big enough to reach the pedals and pounding down on them to get the roll turning and producing music ranging from Scott Joplin to Chopin.

I was absolutely bewitched by the process and would listen to the music for hours at a time. When I got tired of this, I would play the piano by ear, trying to remember some of the tunes I had been taught during my piano lessons at Nazareth House. Another magical item in the room was a brand-new combined stereophonic record player and radio, a twenty-first birthday present for Pat. There were plenty of shiny black long-playing records that varied from Irish traditional music to jazz (which my auntie Pat loved, including Ella Fitzgerald and Dinah Washington).

In those days I wasn't that keen on jazz, but I fell absolutely in love with all the Irish music, particularly listening to the wonderful voice of the tenor John McCormack. One of his albums had a stunning photograph of him on the front cover, where his eyes appeared incredibly beautiful. There were so many songs that I loved, and still do, including, of course, 'The Wearing of the Green'.

There were also records by a singer called Guy Mitchell, and I was to play 'Singing the Blues' repeatedly, along with 'She Wears Red Feathers'. The other one I nearly wore out was 'The Story of My Life' by Michael Holliday. Radio also introduced me to pop music, and I adored Eddie Cochran's 'Summertime Blues' and 'Three Steps to Heaven', Joe Brown and The Bruvvers singing 'A Picture of You' and anything sung by Buddy Holly and Adam Faith. A couple of years later, my records of choice were to be The Beatles' 'Love Me Do' and 'Please Please Me'. I was also starting to become interested in folk music and songs such as 'Dirty Old Town' by The Spinners.

I was very self-sufficient and could occupy myself because there was so much to explore and so much space, having come from Wolverhampton where we were all on top of each other. My other major pastime was reading and it was a joy to be in a household where everybody seemed to be a bookworm. When I was older, it was my responsibility to cycle to the library to return our books. Armed with their list of titles and authors, I would select a fresh batch for Gran, Pat and myself. It was always a pleasure, as it meant I could spend a long time there. The librarians knew me and would take great interest in discussing the books I enjoyed, often suggesting new authors and titles.

Newspapers were part of my reading routine and those delivered to the house included the *Express*. One day I couldn't find the newspaper and hunted everywhere until I discovered it stuffed down the back of the sofa. On the front page was splashed the 1963 Profumo scandal that involved the Tory Secretary of State for War, John Profumo, model Christine Keeler and a member of the Russian Embassy. Fortunately, being a fast reader, I managed to finish the whole article quickly and hide the paper back where it had been originally concealed.

By now I had settled down well with my grandparents and felt safe. I'd left behind thoughts of my mother in Wolverhampton, as it had been such a negative experience; I was protecting myself in a way. I was drawing on the positive as that's my nature; it's something I always do and it's helped me enormously. Being thrown into a new school and a new family at the age of eleven meant I was struck by what was in front of me, and everything was so different and comfortable, I just enjoyed it.

One thing I particularly remember was having a handkerchief – I'd never had one in Wolverhampton. I was always sneezing due to allergies, and there I would have to wipe my nose with my hand. That's an important bit of evidence about the poverty at my mother's: that something so basic wasn't possible because we didn't have enough money. Similarly, learning to routinely take care of myself hadn't happened in Wolverhampton. My mother had been so engrossed in basic survival that there was nobody supervising me washing myself or changing my underpants on a daily basis. The luxury of fresh laundry and a drawer full of clean clothes and underwear was something we didn't have.

I would also flinch at unexpected noises in Wallasey, and it gradually dawned on me that if there was any sort of sudden movement I would put my arms up to protect myself. This was the result of my stepfather physically abusing me. I was slowly learning not to be scared anymore, but Ken did leave a lasting impression on me – even now, I react if anything unexpected happens. That period with him – that gradual build-up to physical abuse – has scarred me. I detest violence now and it scares me. I hate to see children hit and have intervened once, which I wouldn't normally do. It was in a supermarket and a mother slapped her child. I just instinctively went over and said, 'Please don't do that.' We actually ended up getting into a decent conversation because my health visitor mode kicked in, and I enabled her to say, 'Oh he's getting on my nerves,' and I said, 'I can understand how hard it can be when you're exhausted and on your own.' She was full of remorse and knew she shouldn't have done it, and the child was looking up at us both with such relief. It definitely comes from that experience with Ken.

Chapter 15:
School Days

One of the first challenges facing my grandparents was that my eleven-plus exam results had somehow gone missing between Wolverhampton and Wallasey. There was great consternation, as I was due to start secondary school in three months and the results would determine whether I went to a secondary modern or grammar school. As Auntie Pat recalled: 'So, my dad stirred things up and as far as I know, they sort of said, look this child's got to know where she's going when she moves from junior school and we haven't got much time, so get your finger out and do something about it. Because they weren't sure whether you'd passed the eleven-plus or not, they put you into Wallasey Technical High School.'

The all-girl school turned out to be ideal, and it was an extremely happy time for me, although it was all a bit scary to start with. On the first morning, I was accompanied by my grandmother. I have a vivid picture of entering the playground with her and being overwhelmed at the sight of so many girls who seemed amazingly tall and adult.

Each morning I would enjoy walking the short distance to my friend Mary Parry's house, where I waited for her to finish her breakfast before we set off for school together. As an only child, she was doted on by her parents and fussed over by her mother, who made sure she ate everything. Her mum was very kind and always offered me a cup of tea and would chat away with the pair of us. My best friend was Jennifer Salisbury, aka 'Salty', who was an excellent athlete and great fun to be with.

Every four years or so, all the pupils and staff would gather to pose for a school photograph. My original one was lost decades ago but, courtesy of Facebook, I recently managed to find a copy. Taken in 1960 during my second year, it's clear to see that I'm the only Black pupil in the entire school. Sitting next to my neatly dressed friend Mary Parry, my appearance is more akin to that loveable scruffy hero of Richmal Crompton's famous *Just William* books. My hair looks unkempt (I didn't possess an afro comb in those days), my tie is askew and I am squinting at the camera. It wasn't long after that the French teacher realised I couldn't see anything on the blackboard and I was diagnosed as being very short-sighted.

How my grandparents explained me to strangers or the neighbours is a mystery to me now. According to my auntie Pat: 'When you went to the Technical High School, being the only Black kid in the school, I think you got a bit spoiled. I mean, that was only my impression, but you got away with murder, basically. I remember you saying once that somebody got told off for doing something and you'd done exactly the same and they didn't tell you off, you know. But no, I think, as far as I remember, you quite enjoyed the Tech. You weren't somebody who was looking for people to help you with your homework particularly. You seemed to cope with all that yourself.'

This is a thread that seems to go through my life, because I thought I was spoiled at Nazareth House, too. There's a very funny joke by mixed-race comedian and presenter Trevor Noah, when he talks about being small in a white environment and everyone saying, 'Isn't he gorgeous?' Then his Black friend arrives and that becomes all too much for the white folks.

Even though I was cheeky and a bit naughty, I was intelligent and liked being with adults and would have engaging conversations. For a long time, I'd have been the only Black child they ever would have met and I wasn't perceived as a 'threat'. Even for me, it was only a very gradual realisation in my teenage years that my skin colour would have an impact on me, my family, my friends, and it was very minimal.

The school provided me with a sound academic education alongside fantastic sporting activities. Apart from white shirts and socks, the colour of our uniform was green – skirts, summer dresses and the most unbelievable baggy green knickers. We were each allocated to a school house, all named after famous women such as Edith Cavell and Mary Slessor, and each had their own coloured tie. Mine was to be Helen Keller, and our tie was green.

Although I have managed to mislay all of my school reports, courtesy of my cousin Anne I have a copy of a letter written on 12 December 1958 by our grandfather to her father, my uncle Michael, who was serving in the merchant navy. He always looked so handsome in his uniform and would ultimately rise to be a captain of his own ship. I would have been at Wallasey Technical High School for three months when Granddad wrote: 'Elizabeth seems to be getting along OK at school and has got an A for Maths (in which I can claim a share) and is expecting an A for French (no thanks to me, but Pat helps a bit).'

He also notes that 'Mama and Elizabeth are going over to see Mary at Wolverhampton on Sunday, so Pat will have to be the chef.' (I have no recollection of travelling with Gran to see my mum, or of any visits she made to Wallasey to see me. Then again, there are so many things I have forgotten, but it is strange that I can remember her visiting me as a young child at Nazareth House convent.) The letter demonstrates Granddad's affectionate nature in this sign-off to his son: 'Cheerio for now, Michael, love from all at home. Looking forward to seeing your smiling face in the very near future.'

A few weeks later was Christmas and Uncle Michael and his wife, Doreen, who was now pregnant with their first child, Sean, came to stay. (Born the following year, Sean was the sweetest little boy and I would take a great deal of pleasure entertaining him when he came to stay. As a toddler, his favourite pastime was when I perched him on the front gate so that he could shout out whenever he saw a car or a bus.) The dining room was decorated and we all sat around the large table to eat a wonderful dinner. Uncle Michael had bought me some mechanical wind-up toys from Hong Kong – how I adored them. I was also given books (including a much-loved copy of *Old Possum's Book of Practical Cats* by T. S. Eliot), jigsaws and clothes – it was a Christmas I would never forget.

At school, my favourite subjects were French, English literature, geography, biology and history, and I was to pass them all at O level, as well as English language and maths. I absolutely loved French and my French teacher. My mother was obviously brilliant at learning languages and I inherited some of her ability, as I could speak French really well but was less good when it came to grammar and writing. My French teacher used to turn a blind eye to my written pieces because I wasn't shy of talking in the language, which teachers must like in their students.

I was a very fast reader and one day this caused me some embarrassment. Our English teacher had issued the class with brand new copies of *Pride and Prejudice* by Jane Austen and brown wrapping paper, instructing us to cover the book and bring it back the next day. Before the lesson had started, I told a friend that it was a fantastic novel. 'Miss, Miss!' she shouted out, 'Elizabeth says she read the whole book last night!' As we were filing out of the class, the teacher asked me to stay behind and asked a few questions about the novel. While initially mortified, I managed to answer her questions correctly. On escorting me out of the room, she said well done and patted me on the back. Although pleased, I secretly vowed never to allow such an incident to happen again. (It is still one of my favourite books of all time, though!)

Maths had started off well, as can be seen from my granddad's letter. Unfortunately, we then seemed to have a teacher who failed to keep my attention and I started to lag behind. Many of us began to hate maths until a wonderful new teacher arrived. She started off by stating that most of us would fail the GCE exam if we didn't pull our socks up. After a discussion with us about our problems, she gave us the most incredible pep talk ever and committed to working as hard as she could to help us. More importantly, her teaching methods were marvellous as she steered us through seemingly impenetrable problems. Our confidence restored, we were then able to start thinking for ourselves. I thought she was a great educator, and this was proved when many of us *did* pass the exam.

My teacher also introduced me to a couple of new hobbies. One was chess, which I played during the school lunch break, and the other, via her husband, was collecting matchbox labels. He gave a talk about his hobby, phillumeny, and I was entranced; soon I, too, became an enthusiastic collector, otherwise known as a phillumenist ('lover of light'). It wouldn't take long before I accumulated several albums of matchbox labels from all over the world. The box needed to be soaked in water in order to peel off the label and, once dried, pasted into an album.

I joined the Phillumenist Association and was then able to correspond with people in far-flung corners of the world and exchange labels. The letters would arrive with beautifully coloured stamps on them from around the globe, including Russia. This might have raised a few eyebrows, as it was the Cold War era when the West was petrified of a possible nuclear war and the threat from the 1962 Cuban Missile Crisis had been played out across newspapers and the radio. To this day – and I don't know if it was a dream or whether it really happened – I recall an image of huge planes flying overhead against the sky.

Back at school, it became clear that I was ridiculously cack-handed and, as a result, often struggled with art, domestic science and needlework, managing to get thrown out of the latter two classes. Part of domestic science involved various activities in a purpose-built flat, where we were taught to make beds, cook and clean. One day we had been left on our own for a short while and I started to muck around and do handstands on the bed. So I was upside down, balancing against the wall, skirt having fallen over my head, revealing a pair of brown legs and baggy green knickers. Unbeknown to me, in walked both the teacher and headteacher, accompanied by some dignitaries.

Needlework was incredibly difficult, and I was always far behind my classmates in whatever garment we were supposed to be making. One day we had to model our latest item of clothing (which happened to be pyjamas) to some sort of audience. I hadn't managed to complete the sewing and so had just tacked them together but not very well. Sniggers greeted my appearance as the gaping holes showed sections of my skin. I also had to hold up the pyjama bottoms, as there had been insufficient time to insert a cord into the waist area.

While, thankfully, I was removed from these classes to double up on other more enjoyable ones, these mishaps never seemed to get me into serious trouble with any of the teachers. I can't remember any diabolical encounter with a teacher; in contrast, it was more a case of being on the receiving end of a lot of encouragement and good humour.

From being stunned and quiet on my arrival to making friends and feeling safe, I had settled down, but it wasn't to last. Fifteen months after I arrived, my grandfather had a heart attack. He collapsed at work and was admitted to the nearby David Lewis Northern Hospital in Liverpool. At first, he seemed to be on the road to recovery, but nearly two weeks into his stay, he died in his sleep on 6 August 1959. I didn't go to the funeral but heard many years later that my devastated mother did attend, looking exhausted, having travelled on the very early 'milk' train. Auntie Pat didn't see her again for another eleven years, at Gran's funeral in 1970.

Chapter 16:

Changing Times

After my grandfather died, things slowly began to change. My grandmother had always been very loving, but around the age of fourteen or fifteen, I gradually became aware that she was becoming forgetful and also very difficult. She would repeat information she'd already told you and you'd have to pretend it was the first time you'd heard it.

Both Auntie Pat and I realised that, often, she would be talking to me but not to Pat, or equally the other way round. You'd be walking on eggshells because she could just lose her temper or shout for no reason. She'd make up silly rules and then forget all about them. Looking back, I think she was depressed and irritable and was probably suffering from early onset dementia.

She'd had a history of poor health due to conditions caused by pernicious anaemia and a weak heart – and it's lodged in my mind that in the early days (so the story goes), her treatment for the anaemia included eating raw liver sandwiches. Gran's sense of loss and isolation must have been exacerbated due to Granddad having always taken responsibility for so many aspects of the household. I always thought they were well off, coming from my experience in Wolverhampton, and I didn't know for ages that Pat, who was working as an accountant, was having to pay the mortgage now. I'd assumed they'd bought the house.

As a teenager, I had no idea what the matter was, and to me she'd just become a right old nagging so-and-so; I probably wasn't very sympathetic. It shows what ageing, illness and widowhood can do to a person. Fortunately, my relationship with Pat was excellent and we used to love going cycling together. It was a huge thrill when I got my very first bike, a second-hand red one from a shop that was just next door; the owner was always happy to help me out with any problems.

Pat and I would often go out for bike rides. She recalled one interesting episode:

> We were out on our bikes on the promenade near New Brighton. We had a break and sat on the bench and this elderly lady trotted along and sort of nodded and smiled, and we smiled back. Then she got into a bit of a conversation and she said to you, 'You must find it very cold compared to where you're from?' And you said, with your Midlands accent, 'Oh no, it's not as cold as Wolverhampton!' Then you and I nearly had hysterics, only we were too polite, so she trotted on, and she was taken by surprise. She took it for granted you were from abroad because there just weren't any Black people around here at all.

I also still loved phillumeny, which was a suitable escapist pastime, as I was increasingly confined to home on the evenings and weekends; my gran becoming progressively preoccupied with keeping an eye on me. Much later on, I discovered that she was petrified I would follow in my mother's footsteps by meeting a boy and 'getting into trouble'. Even so, I discovered that a fellow phillumenist lived quite near Central Park, and would visit him and his wife and play with their baby.

I also learned that there was a Nazareth House nearby in Birkenhead, and would cycle over to help the nuns on a Saturday afternoon. I recently found a photograph of the children who were there – it reminded me how I've always loved playing with and looking after children. I can see the vulnerability, joy and humour in their faces.

My grandmother also signed me up to clubs run by the local Catholic Church, the first being the Girl Guides – it was fun doing all the activities required to obtain the various badges. There was also a camping trip, which (apart from singing round the campfire) wasn't particularly enjoyable. I woke up exhausted and wheezing due to the cold, lumpy ground and having been petrified of the cows mooing in the adjacent field. One evening there was an international extravaganza at the town hall; we were issued with a flag and then proceeded up to the platform. I was somewhat bemused by being issued with one from an African country because the patrol leader said I 'looked the part'.

The other group I was obliged to attend was the Children of Mary. We had to listen to boring talks by nuns and were told that as Catholics, we were better than those who prac- tised other religions. Once, I challenged this and pointed out that as children didn't choose their religion, they shouldn't be penalised just because they happened to be a Protestant, Buddhist or Muslim. This was not taken to kindly and I was told to be quiet. So I started playing truant and visited my phillumenist friend and his family instead, until my grand- mother was eventually informed about my absences.

It probably didn't help my relationship with Gran that, during this period, I ceased to believe in the existence of God. My reading was wide and varied and, at some point, the local parish priest discovered me with a book by Somerset

Maugham. I was informed that it was on the *Index Librorum Prohibitorum* ('List of Prohibited Books') that Catholics were banned from reading. When replying that I wasn't aware of this, I was told it wasn't possible to know what was on the list. It was all quite farcical; fortunately, the Index was discontinued in 1966.

As it became clear that I was losing my faith, Gran decided to send me off to a Catholic retreat in Liverpool. I was the youngest person in attendance and a monk asked me why I was there. I poured out my heart to him concerning my difficulties in believing there was a God and the various methods I had used to try to prove there was indeed one. This included goodness knows how many recitations of the rosary and looking for a sign from the statue of the Virgin Mary. Having been well and truly indoctrinated in my early life, I would hope to see blood flowing from her heart or some such miracle. The monk started to smile and said that I should stop worrying, and that my faith may or may not be restored in the future. Then he asked if I wanted to go back home and burst out laughing when my quick-fire response was 'No!' It was like a holiday for me, as I was away from my gran's near-constant nagging. He really went up in my estimation when he not only allowed me to stay, but also promised to have a word with our parish priest.

I would often go to Liverpool to stay with my great-aunts (sisters of my grandfather). Kate had been a teacher and Lil a seamstress, and they lived in the West Derby area of the city. Although they seemed incredibly old and extremely religious, I was surprised at how much good fun they were. They taught me to play the card game canasta, and I was taken aback when one accused the other of cheating until I realised they were smiling. One incident has remained etched in my memory: we were out walking and met one of their neighbours. I was amazed when one of my great-aunts introduced me as a child who had been adopted by my grandparents. It gave me a lot of mixed feelings: on the one hand, there was shock and humour that such a devout Catholic person was openly lying and, on the other hand, such sadness that they couldn't tell the truth about me. I began to understand that my skin colour was a cause of shame to them and there was no way they were going to discuss the truth of who I was – my mother's daughter – with anyone, or admit that I was a relative of theirs.

The other holiday I remember was a cycling one to Llandrindod Wells in Wales, organised through our local church. We were a bunch of male and female teenagers and it was my first real contact with boys. I was very shy and kept away from them as much as possible, having a great time with the girls instead. These were welcome breaks from what was becoming an increasingly gloomy time at home.

As I grew older, I would take myself off to watch films on a Saturday afternoon. One that transfixed me was *The Quiet Man* starring John Wayne and Maureen O'Hara. Set in Ireland, it had the added bonus of all the brilliant Irish music that was played throughout the film. It even included 'The Rakes of Mallow' as the backdrop score to the famous fight scene. I stayed on to watch it a second time, and on exiting the cinema bumped into Pat and her boyfriend (later husband) Alex. She warned me that Gran wouldn't be too happy with me. It was worth the risk, though.

There were increasingly severe restrictions on my activities and I wasn't allowed to go to the youth club. This was the era when The Beatles performed locally in New Brighton and the Twist was all the rage. (Years later, my friends could not believe that I couldn't do the iconic dance. They instructed me to pretend that I was drying the top of my back with a towel while stubbing a cigarette out with my foot. Sadly, I never quite mastered it . . .) Gran also insisted that I had to go to bed at 7.30 p.m. every night and that the light had to be switched off promptly; she would tell me off if she caught me using a torch to read a book under the blankets.

A couple of years after I arrived in Wallasey, Pat started going out with Alex, a South African who worked in the Vauxhall car factory in Ellesmere Port. They'd met at a New Year's Eve dance in New Brighton, becoming engaged in 1962, and were married in October 1963 – the first wedding I ever attended. While I remember being delighted with a home-made orange dress, the group wedding photo shows me in the back row, looking anxious and peering out between Pat and Gran. Perhaps it was a portent of what was about to transpire.

Following their marriage in Wallasey in October 1963, Pat and Alex travelled to Ireland for a week's honeymoon and it was at this time that my gran dropped a bombshell: I would be returning to my mum and Ken's in Wolverhampton immediately. I presumed that her decision was due to my 'bad behaviour' of staying out without permission with a friend in Central Park until 5.30 p.m., playing truant from the Children of Mary and my increasing lack of faith.

Worst of all, I had been in the lower sixth for only a few weeks and was enjoying it immensely. The teachers knew that my heart was set on becoming a nurse but often told me that I was university material. When the head teacher heard from my gran that I'd be leaving, she and my beloved French teacher came to visit her to plead my case. I was so touched by this and the fact that they tried their best to comfort me during my utter sense of shock and desolation at this awful news.

To my surprise, Pat later told me that I was being sent away for a completely different reason:

> When I got married and went to Ireland on honeymoon, I didn't know you would be leaving and you'd gone when I got back. Nobody had told me, and I got the impression that because Alex was a white South African, my mum thought that he wouldn't want to live with a Black child in the house. I don't know. She never said anything to me. It was presented to me as a fait accompli. She said you'd gone to do a nursing course. I mean, as far as I knew, that was that. I rather gathered when you got older that she'd thought that it might cause friction, which I don't think it would have.

I would never see my gran again. Unbeknown to me, she died in February 1970, while I was living in Paris; I only found out a few years later.

Chapter 17:

Sudden Departure

Once again, I can't remember the journey back to Wolver-hampton at the age of sixteen. Possibly, I was in a dreadful state of shock. I could have been in a rage as well – I must have felt antagonism towards my grandmother for taking me away from the school that I loved, as well as suddenly having to leave my friends. There would also have been fears about the situation I was returning to in view of the circumstances that led to my departure just five years before.

My mother hadn't been in a position to visit me during the time that I lived in Wallasey and my feelings towards her were now very mixed. On the one hand, she had sent me to a place of safety to get away from Ken's treatment. On the other, she'd not been able to prevent my grandmother from sending me back to a place I now hated with a vengeance. After all, in spite of the later difficulties with my grandmother, I had really loved Wallasey and dreaded the contrast with what life would be like in Wolverhampton.

The family set-up had changed in my absence. Kenny was back with his mother in Bolton, Mick was now ten, Frank six, and there was now Marion (two) and Pam (one). I can't remember the sleeping arrangements exactly – presumably the boys were in one of the bedrooms and Pam was with her parents, and there is a vague memory of bunk beds in the smaller third bedroom for Marion and myself.

There was no question of my returning to school, so my first priority was to get a job. Part of me wanted to go to work and contribute – I wanted to help my mother. I didn't feel resentful, because I'd never planned to go to university and having left a school that I'd really loved, starting a new lower sixth was just not going to happen. Plus, I knew I wanted to be a nurse; this was just a waiting period before I could start at eighteen. Ken immediately came into his own, as he was very familiar with the process of looking for jobs, following habitual altercations with various bosses. It was an era of virtually full employment in many parts of Britain and he was keen to take me to the jobcentre. He looked on proudly when I answered questions about my educational qualifications, and we both noted the look on the interviewer's face when my seven GCE O level subjects were set out. With my desire to be a nurse, I was immediately found a post as a school nurse assistant at Park Lane Infant Welfare Clinic.

Fortunately for me, the clinic was within close walking distance of the house in Low Hill. It was the very same one from which, five years or so earlier, I had picked up the dried infant milk and orange juice for my brother Frank. My duties were to assist the qualified school nurses and to help out with any other work that was needed. It was an enjoyable time and I seemed to get on with all of the staff, although it wasn't without hiccups – for example, when operating the small telephone switchboard, I managed to cut off a call to one of the doctors. Fortunately, no one got cross, but I was never asked to do this task again. My very first pay packet contained notes and cash in a small brown envelope, and I felt like a proper adult. I used it to buy a set of cutlery and crockery for my mother, as I was appalled at the grotty knives and forks in the house.

I started to apply to London teaching hospitals to train as a nurse, including St Bartholomew's (aka Barts), St Thomas' and Great Ormond Street Hospital for children. All the application forms required a photograph of yourself, plus details of your father's name and occupation, which I had left blank – there was no way I was going to ask anyone about him.

The medical officer at the clinic where I worked thought highly of me and would ask me, 'Have you heard back?' One day he grew impatient over the whole thing and said, 'What's the matter with them? You'd make a really good nurse.' It really boosted my confidence, but there wasn't one acknowledgement from the hospitals, in spite of my decent exam results.

Looking back on the lack of response, I think it was a class thing more than anything – teaching hospitals thought they were a cut above general district hospitals. They were for the daughters of surgeons and people with connections, like so many other things in Britain. I've since met Black individuals who trained at teaching hospitals, but there was a snobbishness associated with the institutions – historically, it was daughters of African diplomats and princes who would be accepted. (Kofoworola Abeni Pratt, who is often erroneously referred to as the first Black nurse to work in the NHS, was the daughter of a prominent Nigerian family; there had been people from across the Commonwealth who had worked in medicine in Britain well before the NHS was set up in 1948.)[1]

In response, the medical officer advised me to write off to his alma mater teaching hospital, St Mary's in Paddington, and told me that he'd give me a reference. By mistake, I applied to the nearby non-teaching hospital, Paddington General in Harrow Road, and was immediately invited for an interview.

Travelling there with my mother, it was my first taste of London (maybe for her, too), and the long and bustling Harrow Road was full of shops and people. This was in the early 1960s and I couldn't believe the huge Black migrant presence, plus all the other ethnic groups, as well. Black, brown and white, seeing people who looked like me . . . back in the Midlands, I was the only one, so what struck me was, 'Wow, this is so diverse.' I had a sense of excitement: this was something different and it was exactly what I wanted.

My mother – I was asked to bring an adult with me – sat in on my interview with the matron and a couple of other women, and we learned that I'd been accepted. The three-year State Registration Nursing course would start in September 1965, when I would be eighteen years of age. I couldn't wait. My mother and I would never have discussed what she felt about me following my dream, but she was always encouraging. We never had fireside chats – it was all about survival. She was working and I was trying to stay out of Ken's way.

Chapter 18:

A Place of Safety

Back in Wolverhampton, the stress of living with my mum and Ken in a cramped, damp house where both adults were heavy smokers had started to affect my health. My asthma became worse, exacerbated by the dreadful pea-souper fogs. Wolverhampton remained a very industrial city and it was still common to see smoke billowing from the tall chimneys of many factories in the area. One day there was a particularly nasty fog, but although I was feeling unwell and wheezing quite badly, nothing would stop me from going to work. The fog was so dense that it was only possible to see a yard or so ahead, so you had to put your arms out in front of you to feel your way, which was quite frightening.

Coughing and spluttering, I carried on, as the clinic was nearby. All of a sudden, a man put his hand on my shoulder and asked me what was wrong. I was unable to answer him due to being so breathless. When he proceeded to lead me into Park Lane Clinic, I tried to explain that this was my workplace, but he hushed me, saying that he was a doctor. While my asthma attack was being treated I could hear hushed voices discussing my home situation. The staff were obviously very concerned about me, and it was decided that I would be transferred immediately to work as a school nurse assistant at Kingswood, a residential open-air school for delicate children in Albrighton, on the border with Shropshire. While close to Wolverhampton, it was in a rural area and near to RAF Cosford. Three years earlier, in 1960, the school had moved half a mile to purpose-built premises, so at the time of my arrival it was virtually brand-new. It was run by Wolverhampton Education Authority in collaboration with the local health authority.

The children had a variety of chronic conditions such as asthma, heart ailments and cerebral palsy. There is no record of when I moved to this new job, but it was probably just a few months after starting work at Park Lane Clinic. I have never forgotten this act of compassion towards me by those managing the child health services. Their intervention helped me enormously during this traumatic phase of my life, and I stayed for nearly two years before going to London to study as a nurse at the age of eighteen. It was a wonderfully cathartic interlude, because everything was comfortable and everybody was very kind and easy to get on with. It was a self-contained community that felt secure, and I could see my short-term future mapped out quite clearly. It's something I've always appreciated and feel incredibly lucky to have experienced.

For the first time, I felt truly independent and I savoured every minute of it. My role was once again to assist school nurses, the older of whom was also a resident. My immediate boss was a younger nurse who seemed more like a model; her husband was a racing driver. There was also a cleaner who always wore a gingham overall. She loved to have a good old gossip and was pleased to see that I listened to every word of her tittle-tattle. While I was initially in awe of the younger nurse, she and all the other staff were very helpful and friendly.

I was to care for whichever children had been admitted to the sick bay and I loved looking after them. This included making beds, bathing, toileting and giving the children their meals. One pupil I remember was a young South Asian girl with moderately severe physical and learning disabilities due to cerebral palsy. Always smiling and laughing, she was an absolute delight to look after. With more experience, I was taught how to do inhalations and take temperatures. We would also go across to the main school to inspect the children's hair for nits and lice. It was no surprise to be called 'Nitty Nora, the Great Explorer'.

The authorities organised for me to attend a one-year day-release pre-nursing course at a college in Wolverhampton. This was another agreeable experience, where I was to make friends and learn first aid and human biology – as well as thoroughly enjoying the incredibly good chips that were on offer in the local canteen.

At Kingswood, I was allocated a lovely bed-sitting room in the medical building that housed the sick bay, which was adjacent to the school block. To have such wonderful accommodation was an absolute luxury. For the first time, I was independent from my family, earning a wage and also in a safe place.

That's what I really remember, having money – my rent was taken out of my pay packet and everything else was just for me. From my weekly wage, I saved up to buy books and my very first record player, a Dansette, which was all the rage at the time due to the reasonable cost. It was possible to stack and play several records, one after the other. The first singles I bought included my favourite singers Bob Dylan, The Rolling Stones, The Supremes and the Liverpool folk group The Spinners. I also bought classical records such as

Beethoven's Piano Concerto No. 5 'Emperor' and the music for the ballet *Giselle* composed by Adolphe Adam. I would cheerfully blast out the music to my heart's content. I also remember being surprised to see how many pairs of stockings belonging to another member of staff were hanging out to dry. I asked whether they all belonged to her, and when she said yes, I decided that it might be a good idea to buy a few more for myself – I'd been so used to making do with very little.

The headmaster, Mr Frank Macmillan, and his wife and twin adult children lived in the head teacher's cottage that was down a little lane around the corner from school. A long drive led up to the entrance of the school and we could see it from the medical block, so it was easy to see when Frank (as everybody called him) arrived, motoring up the driveway in his beloved green Austin Mini Countryman, with those distinctive wood inserts in the rear body of the car. Tall and walking with a stoop, he was a gentle giant and a wonderful teacher.

Everybody was friendly and I remember being invited to the home of a younger member of staff who lived on a local farm. Lunch consisted of a buttered roll containing cheese and apple, a combination I had never encountered before but which turned out to be extremely tasty; I was being opened up to other worlds. I can't remember ever visiting my mother and family in Wolverhampton during this period; I didn't want to be in contact with them, and harboured feelings of anger and resentment towards both her and Ken.

Meanwhile, at Kingswood I became very independent as well as quite adventurous – characteristics that were to remain with me over the years. Salty was one of the few school friends from Wallasey I'd kept in touch with. In the summer of 1965 (just before I moved to London), we went on the first of four consecutive annual holidays together, one in Cornwall, one in London and two overseas. In Cornwall, we travelled all the way down to Land's End. I still have some lovely photos of us both at that time. Lack of money was no hindrance, as hitch-hiking was our mode of getting to wherever we wanted to be. It didn't seem as hazardous for eighteen-year-olds as it might today, and it was a fairly common sight back then.

We always stayed in youth hostels, and there was a very puritanical view about how we were supposed to travel (healthily hiking from one establishment to another), so we would ask to be dropped off within reasonable walking distance and then pretend to huff and puff our way to the reception. We became skilful liars when comparing details of our itinerary with the more serious walkers who would also be spending the night at the hostel. In exchange for an incredibly cheap overnight stay, we were rightly expected to take part in the rota of cleaning duties. We would generally sleep in large dormitories on bunk beds, tucked into our sleeping bags. This was when I became aware of my snoring habit, due to often being shaken during the night by an exhausted individual desperate for some sleep. In the end, I would just warn people, apologise in advance and suggest that they stuff something into their ears. It was only during my first year as a student nurse that it was discovered that I had a major blockage in one nostril that required surgery.

Another holiday I undertook, this time by myself, was to cycle from Kingswood all the way through Shropshire to a convent in Llandrindod Wells in Wales. This was in order to stay for a week with my great-aunt Kate, who was now living there since the death of her sister, Lil. Looking back, the whole venture seems a bit crazy, but thank goodness for youth, as it never entered my head that I would encounter any problems. It was a distance of around eighty miles, and I remember cycling along the banks of the beautiful River Dee.

All seemed to be going well until I noticed that it was starting to become so dark that, even with the front light of the bike on, it was impossible to see what was in front of me. Suddenly, I jumped out of my skin when I bumped into something soft, followed by the sound of bleating from goodness knows how many sheep. After shooing them away, I looked around and was relieved to see lights on in a nearby building. Having slowly edged myself towards it, I knocked at the front door and was greeted by a gentleman who told me he was a farmer. When I told him what had happened, he called his wife over and they both started to laugh, while reassuring me not to be worried.

They said I was very close to Llandrindod Wells, but that it was far too late for me to try to cycle there, and that they would put me up for the night free of charge. His wife gave me some delicious hot soup and then showed me to my bed, which I needed to climb up to. It turned out to be one of the best night's sleep that I ever had, due to the most incredibly soft mattress. Next morning, the farmer's wife woke me and brought me up a cup of tea. She later showed me to the bathroom, where there was the most enormously deep bath that I have ever seen, into which she poured hot water from a large jug. After my bath, I was invited to join them for breakfast, and they wanted to know more of my adventures. They said I was one of the funniest people they'd met in a long time and wished me well on the last leg of my journey.

The farmer drew a map of the route to Llandrindod Wells and, as a result, I arrived at the convent in less than an hour.

This was long before the era of mobile phones, and my poor great-aunt had been frantic with worry. I don't think that I had even made a note of the convent's telephone number. My return journey passed without incident except for the onset of short bouts of excruciating acute pain, shooting halfway down my left leg. It lasted on and off for over three decades but, fortunately, this wretched problem disappeared as suddenly as it came on.

The two or so years I spent at Kingswood passed by very quickly without any negative experiences whatsoever. While very sorry to leave, I was really excited to be moving to London to start training as a nurse. My new trunk was packed with all my worldly possessions, a new suit had been bought and I was ready for the big city.

Chapter 19:

Finding My Feet

My life as a student nurse began in September 1965, when I arrived at the nurses' home of Paddington General Hospital in north-west London. Twenty years on, I would discover that the grave of Mary Seacole, the Jamaican-Scottish Crimean War nurse – an icon who would play such a fundamental role in my own life – was less than a mile down the road. Back then, I knew nothing about her, and she wasn't mentioned once during my entire training.

I have a photo taken from my first day with seven of the twelve new nursing students, in which I'm proudly wearing my brand-new suit. Looking at that image, we appear quite fuddy-duddy for eighteen-year-olds. We all had to live in the nurses' home for our first year and, to start with, I was happy living in the small room on an upper floor of the building. There was just enough space for a bed, cupboard, desk and chair, and I found room for my beloved Dansette record player by placing it on top of my trunk. The toilets and baths were further down the corridor. There was a call box on the ground floor, and if you were lucky someone would be passing by when the phone rang. They would rush up and bang on your door and shout out that you had a call. Then it was a matter of running downstairs as fast as you could, hoping that the person was still on the line.

In the other nurses' home near Ladbroke Grove, there was a significant group of students recruited from Hong Kong and Singapore, and the hospital ensured they had an area for Chinese cooking with woks.

A dragon of a woman (a former nurse) was in charge of the home, and she took great pride in keeping a steely eye on our whereabouts. Fortunately, there was a fire escape and some of us came to know it quite well (a third-year student had advised us how to keep it slightly ajar). This came in handy when the front door was locked and we needed to creep back into our rooms in the early hours of the morning.

Paddington General Hospital had been established in the nineteenth century with links to the local workhouse. This might explain the oft-held sentiment that we were seen as the poor sister to St Mary's Teaching Hospital in Praed Street, although the two institutions merged in 1968. (By then, I had qualified as a nurse and would only stay for a further six months or so. Renamed St Mary's Hospital, Harrow Road, it ceased operation in 1986 and the buildings were pulled down and replaced with flats.)

In those days most nurse education programmes were undertaken in a school of nursing that was part of a hospital (and not a university, as is the case today). We studied for three years to obtain our State Registered Nurse (SRN) certificate. In the late 1970s, I would undertake a one-year diploma in advanced nursing at Manchester University to bring my qualification up to degree level. This idea hadn't even entered my mind at this point; I was just thrilled to be starting a nursing course at last.

We spent the first three months of our course attending the Preliminary Training School (PTS) with a proportion of it spent observing on the wards. Our small cohort included several overseas students: Rose from Jamaica, Finny from Finland, Barbara from the Caribbean, Peggy from Hong Kong, then Sue, Janet, Jane, Lynne, Helen, Kay and me, who were from across England. This was my first opportunity of living and working with such a cosmopolitan group of people and I enjoyed it immensely.

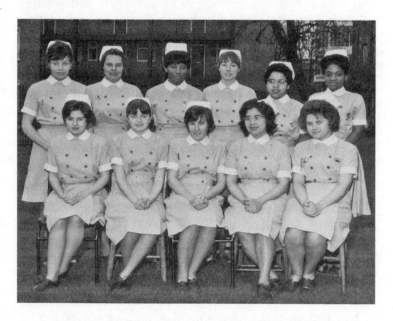

Preliminary Training School, Paddington General Hospital, 1966. I'm in the back row, second from the right.

In this group – Black, white, whatever – we were thrown together for three years. It felt like being back at school and it was very easy to make friends. Rose took me under her wing to try to break down my shyness and, over fifty years later, I'm still friends with Sue and Janet.

Sue reflected:

I remember your keen intellect, which enabled us to have pithy conversations (neither of us liked small talk, although we loved to laugh). [I remember] idealism, left-wing politics, doing the *Guardian* crossword under our desks in PTS lessons, joining the local Labour Party, which was full of coughing, smoking and drinking older men. It's hard to believe now, but I think you found socialising quite difficult in your late teens – the combination of your not suffering fools gladly plus being mixed-race (your 'difference' in other words) alienated you; you seemed English in so many ways but were Black, and I think this confused people and made you stand out. I do remember you talking about going to the convent where the odd nun was cruel to you; your mum and stepfather and how horrible he was to you and how you were left out by him for being Black. I think this engendered in you a sense of not belonging.

Janet also said:

I think the first impression was that you had a good sense of humour, I remember that, and you laughed a lot, but you were not that confident. But you were very English, and I think that's why, somehow, I never saw you as Black. You know, you were just English and I think that's partly because of your accent. You had a very strong mix of Liverpool and Wolverhampton accents, which actually almost identified you really, and perhaps it was that.

We spent a lot of time together in London and what I liked about you, why we got on – you were always game for anything. You would always come with me and if I suggested we should have a curry somewhere, 'Oh yes,' you'd say, 'I'll come.' So whereas you were shy, you had that good sort of spirit – I think that was very noticeable to me – and also the ability to talk about things and understand. There was never anything we couldn't talk about really. I think I would say that to me, you were someone who was very English, who happened to be Black.

This was exactly how I felt, having to this point grown up in a totally white Irish/English culture with no contact or knowledge of my Nigerian roots – everyone, from friends to work colleagues, until I was eighteen was white. Even arriving at Paddington, while I was meeting people from Africa and the Caribbean, there was no one I'd met who was mixed-race or Black British. There were people of my generation who were mixed-race, but they were scattered around the UK. Later, when I was working in Black community projects, other Black people assumed I was from the Caribbean; after all, we all make assumptions about people.

In contrast, I was acutely aware that society viewed and labelled me as 'coloured', 'half-caste' or 'Black'. Talking to Janet and Sue, they saw things that I didn't and were more conscious of my skin colour than I was. They worried for my future – I was naive when I think about it, simply bouncing around and enjoying my life.

Nursing turned out to be better than I had ever hoped. It was the combination of studies, idiosyncratic tutors and, most importantly, caring for patients with an incredible variety of illnesses. My favourite subject throughout training was medical nursing, but most of the other disciplines were of interest, too. Our standard textbook was the 1965 edition of

Toohey's *Medicine for Nurses*, but I can't remember that we were ever encouraged to read articles from journals.

There was a small group of nurse tutors who included Miss Papadopoulos, Miss Dunstan and Mr Adigun. Most of the lectures were quite interesting, although Sue and I were told off for doing a crossword puzzle during a particularly tedious session. Doctors also contributed to the course and I always enjoyed the input of Dr Simon Cohen, a senior registrar who later became a consultant physician in east London. He had a flair for explaining the symptoms of a condition clearly, together with the relevant physiology and anatomy. It was obvious that he enjoyed keeping us awake by a mixture of telling jokes and firing questions at us.

Miss Papadopoulos, or Miss Papa as she asked us to call her, was our sharp and extremely knowledgeable principal tutor. She didn't tolerate ignorance kindly and could be quite caustic when questions weren't answered quickly enough. Having said that, she could occasionally stun us with her wicked sense of humour. Complications of poliomyelitis resulted in her needing to walk with a stick, so we could always hear her approaching the classroom. This was useful for some students who were petrified of her, as she could throw a most withering look when displeased. Fortunately, she took a shine to me and I was awarded the second-year prize. I was allowed to select books up to a certain value, which I still have to this day. They were Philips's *Record Atlas* and Cassell's *French–English Dictionary*, presented to me on 18 October 1967.

The mock-up ward in the school of nursing was also used for medical students' practical examinations. Real patients were brought in for the day and, on several occasions, Dr Cohen obtained permission from Miss Papa for me to help out at the sessions. During one of these times, he asked me to consider studying medicine, adding that he'd be happy to explore this if I was interested.

I didn't have a desire to study medicine; my decision to be a nurse – from the influence of the 'white nun' from Nazareth House onwards – was all about direct contact with patients. While very touched, I explained that nursing was exactly the career for me and that I didn't wish to switch to medicine even though I was capable of it, a decision that I've never regretted.

Chapter 20:

Becoming a Nurse

After Preliminary Training School, we were kitted out in our mustard and white student nurse uniforms in readiness for our first-ever ward experience. We stayed on the ward for about three months and I was delighted that my friend Lynne was on the same placement. In those days, student nurses were part of the actual ward workforce. Apart from study days, our rota mimicked that of the qualified staff, including night duty. As students, we could easily have times of actually being in charge of a ward, which is frightening to look back on now.

We constantly moved to new wards or departments, and these were the scariest periods during those three years of training. The first few days in a new environment were the worst by far. Being shy was a terrible hindrance, as there were so many staff to get to know, never mind the patients. My stomach would be in knots during those first days, so whenever possible I would escape to the sluice and pretend to be busy washing bedpans.

Nursing activities on the ward included bed-making, bathing patients, cleaning lockers, giving out meals, and doing dressings and the drugs round. There was also the regular recording of patients' temperatures, pulses and respiratory rates, together with their blood pressure readings.

If possible, I would keep clear of the doctors' rounds, with all the fuss and pomposity that surrounded most of them.

We nurses were expected to be busy little bees completing all of our tasks, not talking to patients or sitting on their beds, which was severely frowned upon. In those days, they were called Nightingale wards and had sixteen to eighteen beds in them. It posed a major problem for me, because I was so curious. I loved reading the patients' notes then getting to know the people behind them. I had a natural intelligence about me that knew that the more you can find out about someone, the more you could help them.

So whenever the chance arose – the best opportunities arose when giving a bed bath, doing a dressing or accompanying them to the bathroom – I would just ask a few questions and listen to their answers. Even just talking to them about how they liked their tea or boiled eggs, you could see people responding positively because you'd bothered to ask. I remember people saying, 'Normally we just get it plonked in front of us.'

There was the odd ward sister who recognised that I could elicit information from patients. For example, if someone was depressed, I could find out what was worrying them, particularly if they weren't compliant or adhering to treatments. Why would someone not want to do something that would help them get better? Often, it was a case that they were frightened by things or unsure why we were treating them that way.

For example, people lying down in bed can get pressure sores, which is where the circulation stops in a particular area and starts to cut off oxygen. It can lead to the skin breaking down and wounds and necrotic ulcers where the skin dies. So you want to ensure that people get out of bed or roll over so you can massage the area a little when you're giving them a bed bath. But people can often be scared of moving because it might cause them pain and some just 'don't bloody want to move'. So you have to negotiate and they need an explanation why.

This was the era of authoritarian doctors and nurses with subservient patients – people weren't expected to question things and would be called difficult if they did. But they weren't difficult, they were bloody-minded. I liked bloody-minded people, because often there was a good reason why they were that way. I found it in an interesting challenge to break through that; often being polite, respectful, using a bit of humour and giving explanations made all the difference. I knew not only would it help them, but it would also make my job a lot easier. And whether you're on a ward or you're a health visitor, you've got to get around a lot of patients and families; it makes things a lot faster and more efficient, rather than being held up by different scenarios. Most patients poured their hearts out, and I soon became acquainted with a rich and diverse Paddington population.

There was a significant number of Irish patients, and they were usually very surprised to hear of my own origins; some would have me in fits of laughter with their jokes and stories. There was one lady who I'd told that I had Irish relatives. She said in a nice way, 'No. Really? No.' And I said, 'Really – I can even do Irish dancing.' And she said, 'No you can't!' I looked around the ward and there were very few people there, so I did an Irish jig for her. There's a jig where you do one, two, three, four, five, six, seven. One, two, three. One, two, three. And you go across and you go back. She was laughing so much I had to stop, as I was worried in case she had stitches.

In contrast, there was a minority of patients I used to dread having to look after. One was an older woman on an orthopaedic ward recovering from a hip operation that hadn't gone very well. As a result, she had been on the ward for a very long time and seemed to take pleasure in picking out one new student and making their life hell. Unfortunately, I was one such target; once she made me go back to the kitchen three times to boil an egg to her exact standards. I finally refused at the fourth demand. After that bruising experience, I would often speed past her bed, acting as though deaf, blind and dumb – not the best nursing care, of course. It was therefore not a shock when she reported me to the sister who, to my eternal gratitude, listened to my account and had a quiet word with the patient. However, she did give me a few tips on dealing more compassionately with a so-called difficult patient, including discussing issues with experienced staff on the ward.

My weak area was poor manual dexterity (otherwise known as cack-handedness, as I mentioned before). I would envy those nurses who could, for example, speedily and efficiently remove stitches. One surgeon had me thrown out of the operating theatre when I dropped an instrument on the floor. He was quite tall and I had already irritated him by being unable to secure the back of his gown quickly enough. It didn't help that he kept wandering about as I leaped up behind him trying in vain to tie the tapes. He was absolutely right to get rid of me and I was quite pleased, as theatre nursing frightened the life out of me. I hated the arrogance of some of the doctors. There were some who didn't even notice you were there. There was also the male–female imbalance going on, with more male doctors than there are today and more women working as nurses.

While some ward sisters were absolute dragons, most were helpful and some even good fun. The one I was to remember most was in charge of my very first ward. Lynne and I had been told to go and lay out a deceased man under the supervision of a third-year student, who promptly left us to it. It was our first contact with a dead person, and we were both petrified. Peering around the screens surrounding the bed, we both gasped. There was what appeared to be a huge body beneath the sheet, as his abdomen was enormous due to fluid that had collected from complications of his illness.

Our initial job was to wash the body and this entailed turning him over to wipe his back. Lynne and I were on either side of the bed and, as we were both very short, had difficulty working out how we were going to complete this task. We looked at each other with anxiety and then I proceeded to roll him towards Lynne. We suddenly heard what sounded like a sighing noise emanating from the body, which frightened the living daylights out of us. Our immediate reaction was to laugh hysterically, which we knew was totally inappropriate. All of a sudden, the screens swished to one side and the face of the ward sister glared at us.

Silence ensued and we were marched off to the office, where we both burst into tears. Very quietly, she asked who had asked us to perform this duty. The third-year student nurse responsible was called in and, in front of us, was brusquely reprimanded by the sister for not staying with us and supervising everything. Before all three of us went back to complete the unfinished business, I was amazed when she made tea for everybody and chatted about coping with the experience of the death of a patient. Caring for a dying patient would never be easy, but her words of wisdom helped enormously. She explained that it was normal to be frightened of death, and someone did need to explain that to us. Now, you would hope that students would have informal discussions to prepare them and provide a much more emotional approach to issues that would affect them.

It's quite cruel and unthinking to expose naive eighteen-year-olds who had just arrived in London to a dead body with no preparation. Even just to ask, 'Is this your first experience of seeing a dead body?' because it's such a jolt. Thankfully, the ward sister rectified it by talking to us sobbing jellies, reassuring us that we'd done nothing wrong and cleverly and sensitively turning the situation into a tutorial. I've always remembered what that ward sister did and what a useful approach she had in communicating with students, which I've tried to bring into my own teaching.

One other incident that has always stayed with me concerned the searing grief of a bereaved mother. During my final year, I was working in the very busy casualty department when a young adult male was admitted following a drugs-related incident. While being examined, he suddenly collapsed and had a cardiac arrest. The team immediately started trying to resuscitate him but without success, and he was declared dead, much to the shock of all of the staff. He had appeared so physically fit and strong. One of the nurses phoned his mother and I will never forget the sound of her piercing shrieks on hearing of her son's death.

Night duty could be both wonderful and fearful. We would gradually be given more responsibilities during these shifts. Generally, it was less busy, so opportunities arose to spend more time with patients who were anxious and couldn't sleep. Other times, we would be absolutely frantic and just prayed that there was a senior manager available who would actually roll up their sleeves and help us on the ward. Also, that the doctor on call would respect our judgement that, yes, they really *did* need to come now to see the patient. The phone call informing us of yet another admission was what we all dreaded. Tea and meal breaks went out of the window and, in the morning, we were just about able to stagger to the hospital canteen for bacon and eggs. There was something about a gang of you going in together after a shift, knowing you'd see other people you knew. You'd have a giggle and talk things over, and it provided a much-needed psychological support as you talked over what had happened on your shift.

One night, an incident occurred that caused me to get more sleep than I could ever have dreamed of. I was a first-year student and suffering from a particularly severe bout of hay fever. To relieve the symptoms, a doctor gave me a small blue Phenergan tablet, a medicine that I had never taken before. It clearly must have knocked me out, as the next thing I can remember was waking up in my room some twelve hours later.

The group of student nurses I started the course with in 1965 was a small one. As such, we generally stuck together and were fortunately able to share the worst and best experiences of hospital life. We were all away from home (some a long way from home) and we all had that first year in the nurses' home, so there was camaraderie. Plus, we had that dark humour you get in nursing and medicine. I think you probably have it in all professions where you share negative, scary and funny things that happen to you; it's an incredibly good way of releasing tension and sharing knowledge. As eighteen- and nineteen-year-olds, we were all going through big cultural transformations. Sometimes we'd howl with laughter together and sometimes we'd cry over work or our social lives.

After the first year, we were allowed to move out of the nurses' home and quite a few of us couldn't wait for this moment. Four of us rented a flat in Harvest Road that was within walking distance of the hospital. Lynne, Helen, Jane and I were to remain living there until after we qualified and were finally ready to leave Paddington General Hospital.

Chapter 21:

New Horizons

Shyness caused no end of problems during my first year and made me hesitant about going out to socialise. Instead, I would tend to stay in my room and read, play records or listen to the radio. My taste in music was becoming quite catholic, ranging as it did from The Rolling Stones to *Rigoletto*. There was a residents' lounge in the nurses' home where I would occasionally watch television. Above all, one of my favourite pastimes was sleeping. It took me some time to adjust to the physically demanding life of nursing. At times I found the combination of long hours on the wards and revising for exams utterly exhausting. Many years later when I told my friend Sue that I was pregnant, she wondered how on earth I would cope with sleepless nights. She recalled the times when I was off duty, sleeping for up to twenty-four hours following a particularly tiring set of shifts.

My nascent organisational skills came into play at this time, as I got involved in setting up a local student nurses association, probably linked to the Royal College of Nursing. A lasting memory is being invited to visit Germany in March 1968 with a group of student nurses from all over the UK. One photo shows a group of us in blue and white uniforms looking cold outside the entrance of a hospital. Others were taken at Heidelberg Castle, outside Goethe's house in Frankfurt and at a grisly first-aid demonstration in Wiesbaden. We were invited to several official events and I was very impressed that classical music was played during these functions. However, I will never forget my intense embarrassment at a dance we all had to attend, as we were matched up with a male cadet for the evening! In contrast, I thoroughly enjoyed our trips to see other hospitals, although I was shocked at the severe restrictions imposed on parents wishing to visit their small children. They were only able to peer at them through a window of the children's ward.

There were to be other trips abroad during my student days. I was still in touch with Salty, my school friend from Wallasey. In 1966, we hitch-hiked to Switzerland and spent a wonderfully hot day in Lindau on the shores of Lake Bodensee. There was a scary moment while hitch-hiking when Salty dragged me back from a car that was pulling up to give us a lift. Not always known for being observant, I had failed to spot that the driver had exposed himself. The following year, our hitch-hiking adventures took us to Germany, where a less worrying but quite embarrassing incident occurred. A very stern policeman approached and informed us that, unbeknown to the pair of us, we were hitch-hiking illegally on the *autobahn* (motorway). Ordering us to stay where we were, he proceeded to peer at the licence plates of oncoming traffic until a British car approached. To our utter amazement, he ordered the driver to stop and give us a lift. We crept into the back, apologising profusely, but fortunately the driver had a great sense of humour and was not at all annoyed.

One of the few photos taken during this holiday is a lovely one of Salty at Koblenz Castle, overlooking the junction of the River Rhine and River Moselle. This was to be our last trip together, as Salty got married and I sadly lost touch with her.

My final hitch-hiking holiday was with Josephine, a Spanish nursing friend who hailed from Aduna in the Basque province of Gipuzkoa. Her family would have been horrified to know of our travel plans, so we just hitch-hiked across France until we got to the Spanish border. We then took a train to her hometown, where her brothers met us; they remained none the wiser and we managed to have a great holiday in spite of our limited budget. On the way back, my French came in handy when we thumbed a lift in the south of the country from a lorry driver and his mate. I overheard the driver whispering which of us he would go off with when they stopped at a cafe. Poor Josephine had no idea what was going on when I suddenly pretended to retch and double up in pain. The men were clearly astonished that my French was good enough to demand that they stop the lorry so that we could get out. It was only after they had driven off that I could explain everything to her. In 1968, my final year as a student nurse, I took my first flight on a holiday with Sue to a Spanish seaside resort. While not at all fazed by take-off or landing, the bouts of turbulence petrified me and always have ever since. Consequently, I gave up flying in 2005.

Looking back, my social life as a student nurse was torturous at times. I was somewhat frightened of meeting men and was happier going out and having a laugh with our set of student nurses, who all happened to be female. The odd date that I did have never led to a lasting relationship, as one or other of us would finish it after the first or second encounter.

I was in awe of friends like Janet and Sue, who seemed to be so much more at ease in any social setting. Nurses used to organise dances at the hospital and invite policemen from the adjacent Harrow Road police station – I don't know if anybody's ever done a study of how many nurses marry policemen . . . I went to a few of the dances, but didn't enjoy them; in fact, I thought they were awful and so boring. I was very shy and would sit there dreading someone coming to ask me up for a dance I couldn't do.

My friend Janet was a few years older than me and struck me as extremely worldly-wise. She had a lovely car, a small green Mini, and would take me with her on wonderful outings that included shopping sprees. As she relates:

> I had a lot of Chelsea friends and was always wanting to try new fashions, because of course it was that time in the sixties with the miniskirts and things like that, so I did have some white boots and a white hat. I knew you liked them, but I didn't realise how much until the next time I saw you, when you were wearing a pair of white boots and a white hat! It caused me great amusement, because you looked quite incongruous with your black hair and black skin and white boots and white hat, which of course were unseen in Chelsea, and not generally common anywhere in those days.

I wasn't confident about my identity and would express it to my friends. One time, I agreed to go with Janet to a dance in London's Mecca dance hall in Leicester Square, which was quite traditional; goodness knows why, as apart from Irish jigs and reels, dancing was then a no-go area for me. The place was packed and quite overwhelming. At one point, an African man came up to me and said how pleased he was that my hair was natural and asked me for a dance. That was it. I suddenly became quite anxious, said I needed to go to the toilet and just fled the venue without even telling Janet. I couldn't cope with it and felt very insecure. The guy was being really friendly, but I couldn't dance, I was shy around men and Black men, too, despite the fact he had complimented me on my appearance.

Janet's reflections shed light on my behaviour:

> I never thought about you getting married because you didn't seem to like men too much. It wasn't that you disliked men particularly, but you were slightly – I don't know whether afraid is the right word – but timid, unsure. The image that I had of you when I first met you was that you wouldn't have been brave enough to go out with a man, you know, white or Black. I remember you saying, 'Oh, I never want to be with a Black man,' because you never had that connection and they would be alien to you.

I wasn't comfortable with my Black identity and I didn't know Black people. I was scared of Black men, which all makes sense because where was I going to get any positive role models? Plus, I was quite uptight about men.

Not long after this incident, Rose persuaded me to get my hair 'relaxed': in other words, straightened. It's clear from my first passport photo in July 1966 that I still hadn't mastered moisturising and combing my natural hair and, while I was fine with it, until the afro comb came along, my tight, curly hair was difficult to manage. Rose took me to the local Black hair salon for my first experience of the process, which involved using fiery chemicals that burned some of my scalp. While expensive and painful, I liked how my hair looked immediately after a hairdressing appointment, as seen in the photo of me taken as a staff nurse at Paddington

General Hospital (on p.3 of the picture section). My hair would soon become stiff and straight, requiring it to be put in rollers to keep it wavy, and after a few years I became really fed up with it all.

Rose suggested that I accompany her to small parties, organised in the homes of her fellow Jamaican friends. I even went with her a few times to the famous Cue (later Q) Club in Paddington that was run by the late Count Suckle. Friends who noticed how tense I was at social events suggested alcohol could help and this led me to try gin and tonic. It worked for a short period before I started to feel depressed, and someone told me that this was a classic side effect of gin. So I switched to rum and coke, and this suited me better, and certainly helped me to become more relaxed. (Fortunately, I never became drunk, as I didn't enjoy the taste that much, and was able to unwind with just a small amount of alcohol. In addition, the smell of alcohol always reminded me of Ken's drunken antics and rages.)

I fell into the Caribbean house parties much faster than the nurses' dances, which was partly down to the music; I fell in love with it. It was just at the cusp of the end of ska and the beginning of reggae, and they'd play Prince Buster, Peter Tosh, Toots & the Maytals and Desmond Dekker & the Aces, all of which I added to my record collection. It was much easier to dance to and I was no longer one of a few Black faces – everyone was Black. It stopped me from feeling different or that people were looking at me. I've got a lot to thank Rose for – I feel like she took me under her wing.

The late 1960s was a period of unrest in many parts of the world, and there were some that I followed with particular interest. These included the Biafra War in Nigeria (July 1967–January 1970), the May 1968 upheavals in France, the US civil rights movement and the growing international protests against apartheid in South Africa. In the late 1960s, and much closer to home, there was continued police harassment of the West Indi-an-owned Mangrove Restaurant in Notting Hill. It culminated in a demonstration against the police, whose heavy-handed tactics resulted in violence. There followed a well-publicised trial in 1970 of the Mangrove Nine, which included Frank Crichlow, Altheia Jones-LeCointe and Darcus Howe, all of whom were acquitted of the charge of incitement to riot.[1]

On a more personal note, I was very relieved to pass the final exams in October 1968 and become a State Registered Nurse. Unfortunately, a couple of our cohort had to resit their papers. The satisfaction I gained from those hospital nursing days was from making a sick, frightened person as comfortable and reassured as possible, while also trying to understand their condition, treatment and prognosis. Once qualified, I successfully applied for a position as a staff nurse on a medical ward and worked there for about six months. It was a thoroughly enjoyable experience, and the extra responsibilities were a welcome challenge, in a ward that was generally adequately staffed. I was totally unaware that Janet was worried about the impact that racism would have on my future promotion prospects.

> You were doing well in nursing, but I do remember saying to my sister that it's a shame that Elizabeth will never be able to go very far in nursing because of her colour. To my knowledge, I don't know whether this is true, but there didn't seem to be any Black ward sisters and hence the chance of you being one [seemed small].
>
> I mean, we were all aspiring to be ward sisters ulti-mately. I remember when my ward sister was off sick

and I was left in charge of the ward – I was a complete novice, yet we would be in charge of everything. So we were led to believe that ultimately we would be ward sisters. But there was always a thought: well, Elizabeth sadly won't get there.

You came over as being so bright, and I know you got very into politics and were always enquiring and asking questions. I didn't really consciously think about it, but I think society has an impact on us all really, and maybe my feeling was that Blacks were less intelligent than whites. I mean, where would I have got that from? I don't remember thinking that, but society bombards us with this propaganda and therefore to see Elizabeth, you know, Black, but a clever girl, was perhaps different. So therefore I thought what a shame almost – what a shame Elizabeth is Black, because she won't be able to move forwards in her career.

None of this was at all obvious to me at the time, so Janet's comments came as quite a revelation.

The relationship with my mother was probably at its weakest during this period, as I never had any great desire to visit Wolverhampton. I kept in contact via letters, but going home didn't occur to me. Friends were plentiful, nursing was keeping me busy and interested, and I was very happy with my London life.

While having enjoyed the experience of being a staff nurse, I had itchy feet and wanted to move on. In those days it was the done thing 'to do midwifery' after qualifying as a nurse, even if you had no intention to practise as one. So began the process of looking around for a suitable maternity unit. I chose to go to Scotland, as it was a country that had fascinated me since I was a teenager in Wallasey and I had spent many enjoyable hours cutting out a series of Highland figures in kilts from the back of Quaker Porridge Oats boxes.

Chapter 22:

Scotland

My midwife training location of choice was to be the beautiful capital city of Edinburgh. I obtained a place at the Simpson Memorial Maternity Pavilion Hospital, and started in May 1969, on the first one-year integrated midwifery course. Up until then, it was usual to do a six-month Part One course and, if you wanted to become a fully fledged midwife, then proceed to Part Two. There were twelve of us on our course and the cohort photo shows that we were a diverse group. I was to discover quite quickly that the Simpson Memorial Maternity Pavilion was a much more traditional and hierarchical place than what I'd experienced so far.

On our first day, we were issued with a sheet of questions to help us familiarise ourselves with the history and layout of the hospital. The hospital was very proud of the fact that Britain's first antenatal clinic was established there in 1915, and we were tasked with finding some evidence (possibly a plaque) of its existence. However, our priorities on our first day were getting to know each other. We walked down the hospital's long corridors laughing and having great fun, paying no attention to what we were meant to be doing.

As soon as we got back to class and the tutor discovered we'd done no research whatsoever, we got a psychological walloping and were peremptorily sent back to the unit. Oh my goodness, we were like puppies let off the leash and then called back to heel with an angry whistle. The film *The Prime of Miss Jean Brodie* with Dame Maggie Smith had just come out, and this woman was so angry and prim, that's exactly who she reminded me of. We didn't take it too seriously, but it was a wake-up call.

I was struck by the history and hilliness of Edinburgh and I shared a lovely huge flat with some other students in Marchmont Crescent, close to the greenery of Bruntsfield Links and The Meadows. It was a stark contrast to the basic flat I'd lived in at Paddington, which was urban and built-up. Here, there was so much greenery and I loved it – I was starting to realise that, while I adored living in the city, I also appreciated being around the countryside and mountains.

Some of my friends in the cohort included Gerry, Sue and Moggy, and we enjoyed exploring Edinburgh together. This included a dawn climb of Arthur's Seat, which students rudely dubbed as Arthur's Arse. The hill is 822 feet high and overlooks the city. I was still very keen on improving my French, so I registered for lessons at the Institut Français. It was also a must for me to go to the Edinburgh Festival, and I will never forget seeing a magnificent performance by Ian McKellen, in Marlowe's *Edward II*. The play had a shocking end when the homosexual king was killed through having a scorching hot poker put up his backside. It was performed by the Prospect Theatre Company and unsurprisingly caused a storm of controversy.

Back at the Simpson, I was enjoying midwifery, particularly time spent with the women and their babies on the postnatal wards. To start off with, I experienced difficulty understanding those who spoke with a strong accent. One day there was a great deal of laughter when I asked for a 'translation' of the following rapid sentence addressed to me: 'Would you get me a wee goonie [nightgown] for my wee bairn [little baby]?'

There was also a great deal of research undertaken at the hospital. One of our tasks seemed to be forever collecting huge bottles of 24-hour urine samples from the women, without any explanation. The doctors were treated like gods and it was clear that student midwives were at the bottom of the pecking order – no questions were ever encouraged. I can recall that epidurals were still a relatively recent procedure for pain relief during labour. Unfortunately, it went disastrously wrong for one poor woman and, as a consequence, she had been unconscious for some time. All I knew was that she was being nursed in a side cubicle but was never to find out what happened to her.

Student midwives needed to deliver around a dozen babies by the end of their first six months and you had a book to record each case delivery in. Achieving this was not at all straightforward for several reasons. First, as a teaching hospital there were many medical students competing for deliveries. Secondly, it was a major referral centre for women with complex obstetric histories, often leading to a caesarean section or forceps delivery.

Five months or so into the course, I was way behind, so a weird system was developed to address the problem. Those of us in dire need of a delivery were issued with a number. Every so often a midwife would come running into the ward and bellow out a number down the Nightingale ward – it seemed similar to ordering a Chinese takeaway – and if your number came up, you needed to rush out and rapidly follow her down to the labour ward. You'd charge down the corridor together walking really, really fast. On arrival there was barely time to say hello to the mum-to-be before washing your hands and gowning up. Then you would get on with the delivery under the supervision of one of the labour ward staff.

The most appalling incident was when a midwife was actually holding back the head of the baby so that I could deliver it. It was only when it was all over that you could chat to the mother and write up the records and your own notes. The most memorable experience was when I had just delivered a baby and it soon became clear that another, unexpected one, was on its way. Although everyone was caught on the hop, twin two came safely into the world, much to the relief of the mother, me and everyone else. If it wasn't for the poor mothers and babies, it would be funny and a perfect example of where we found dark humour as student midwives. We'd sit there laughing at the farcical system.

Then there were other problems in this hospital: the hierarchical and illogical behaviour of some of the staff was starting to get to me. One day, an older middle-class woman who was both depressed and struggling to breastfeed her baby came onto my ward. I spent some time at her bedside, helping her to relax and telling her not to overanalyse things. She kept blaming herself for the baby not feeding, and she just needed to be talked down from putting so much pressure on herself. When the baby started to breastfeed, it was a huge achievement for her. However, she was exhausted and her depression developed into the more severe mental illness of puerperal psychosis. As a result, she left my ward and was transferred to a psychiatric unit in a different part of Edinburgh. When she recovered she asked her husband, who I remember was a journalist, to contact me and asked if I could visit her. I was so delighted to go to the unit and see how well she was bonding with her child, and cooed over the baby.

However, on my return to the hospital, I was summoned to see the ward sister and shocked when she gave me a dreadful dressing-down. A friend of hers at the psychiatric unit had told her about my visit and she kept furiously repeating, 'Just who do you think you are? Who gave you permission to visit her?' She dismissed my response that I'd been asked to visit by the patient and her husband, which I found both daft and unjust, so it seemed better just to keep quiet. Once out of her office, I struggled to stop the tears from running down my face – I felt she was off her rocker and felt utterly humiliated. I experienced a sense of blackness, both visually and emotionally, surrounding me.

There was no way that I wanted to continue my studies and I decided to look into how to become a health visitor. It meant working outside of a large institution like the hospital, which I now wanted to break out of. I also really enjoyed working with mums, partners and children, trying to help them all, and the feeling that you may be able to contribute more at an individual level. I loved the idea of working in the community and focusing on the health promotion side of public health in order to reduce and prevent illness.

In the meantime, continuing with French classes at the Institut Français helped to lessen my feelings of depression. One day I saw a small announcement on the noticeboard, stating that a family living near Paris were seeking a person to speak English to their two children. My mind was made up: this would be my next move.

A few weeks later, I was walking down the corridor with my head hung low. The hospital matron, Miss Margaret Auld, who was very respected, stopped me in my tracks as she recognised I was no longer the cheerful student she'd seen previously. She said: 'What's the matter with you?' And it was such a powerful question – that didn't have a yes or no answer – that it opened the floodgates for me. She invited me to come into her office, and over a cup of tea and a biscuit which she made for me, she asked me why I had changed so much from the upbeat student of six months ago. I was amazed that she even knew me, never mind the degree of sympathy and support she offered, so I just told her all of my problems.

First, she reassured me, 'You haven't done anything wrong, Elizabeth,' and said she would speak to the sister in question. Then she asked, 'Do you want to be a midwife?' and I was a bit embarrassed to say, 'No,' although many nurses didn't follow that path despite the training. I told her I was hoping to become a health visitor instead. She reassured me that the obstetric experience that I'd gained at the hospital was sufficient to meet the requirements of the course. I would, however, need to find something to do until I could start the health visitor course in the following September. I told her about the job in Paris and she said, 'Go for it.'

Looking back on this incident with the ward sister, I realise now it was bullying and harassment. Since then, I've done talks with midwifery students where their tutor asked me to explore what happened because it has such resonance for anyone who has been bullied – either at work or at school. There are negative and positive aspects to this experience: on the one hand, there was this dragon of a woman being irrational and status-conscious, reminding me I was 'only a student'. She made me feel inferior and powerless just for responding to a request from a patient. Then, on the other hand, there was the matron being kind and enabling me to explain what had happened. All she did was listen – she was at the top of the pyramid and I was at the bottom – but it stopped me from feeling guilty or worrying that I'd broken a rule.

The lesson I take from this is: if you're being bullied, then tell someone. I was lucky that the matron literally stopped me in my tracks, but if you're in a similar position, find someone you can trust who is in a senior position so you can talk it through. You might find that people will support you through that bullying experience, so don't bottle it up and let it cause depression. I was surprised that such a senior person would advocate for a junior person, but it can happen.

When I also think about that mother, I'd do it all again in a flash; it was the humanitarian thing to do. I'm not a woman of faith, but I used to relate to humanism: treating others the way you'd like to be treated yourself. If someone is in difficulty and you've got the expertise or even the time to help them, then it's common sense that you'd do it. Also, it underlines my independent streak – I wanted to break away from hierarchical status-conscious people within the organisation. From my stepfather to this midwifery sister, some people like to exert power over other individuals and it's something I feel incredibly uncomfortable with.

A few weeks later when I heard that the job in Paris was mine, Miss Margaret Auld was one of the first to offer her congratulations and wish me well in France. So in December 1969, at the age of twenty-two, I was about to embark on my first-ever experience of living abroad.

Chapter 23:

Paris

I arrived at the Gare du Nord railway station in December 1969 clutching a photograph of Madame Lacroix. She was co-owner of a maternity and surgical clinic in the Paris suburb of Vitry-sur-Seine, close to Orly Airport. We had exchanged photos, and the plan was that she would collect and drive me to what would be my home for the next nine months. This didn't quite work out, as on my arrival there was a huge crowd and, unfortunately, I wasn't able to spot her in the throngs of people milling about.

After hanging around for a bit, I decided to find a taxi, confident that my French was good enough to communicate the address to the driver. This proved to be the case, but what I hadn't reckoned with was that the trip involved crossing half of Paris. I was staggered at the cost of the fare and thoroughly disheartened at such an expensive start to my stay. Fortunately, Madame Lacroix, who arrived back from the station at around the same time, took pity on me and paid the fare. She was as friendly and as chic as she appeared in her black and white photograph.

We entered the clinic reception and after a few quick introductions to members of staff, took the lift up to the family flat. Once inside, all of the family came to greet me and I was shown around their large apartment that took up a whole floor above the clinic. Both Monsieur and Madame Lacroix were doctors, he an obstetrician and she a neonatologist (a specialist in newborn babies). Monsieur Lacroix was well built, had a Germanic appearance and welcomed me with a smile and a few words of English. It was clear that he adored his wife and that this was a mutually loving relationship. Their son, Jean-Christophe, was ten and their daughter, Martine, eight.

Although my role was principally to help the children with their English, the family were delighted that I spoke some French and could understand them quite well (although the children spoke far too fast for me at times). Jean-Christophe was asked to take me to my room and as we went, chatting in French, he asked me why the British had killed Joan of Arc. Welcome to France! I can't remember my reply, but he appeared satisfied, and we were to get on extremely well during the next nine months. He was a serious, gentle and quiet youngster, and I was really pleased to discover that he had a great sense of humour. Martine was bright, like her brother, very chatty and could be quite feisty at times. She had a great sense of fun and we also got on fine, once I had set a few boundaries and realised that I didn't have to tell them off or be strict because we had so much fun together.

One of the first jokes I played on them was when they asked me to explain a word I had used, namely 'berk' for somebody who was stupid. I said it was too rude to explain and wouldn't let on, despite their pleas, throughout my whole time there or on subsequent visits to see the family. However, eventually I caved in on a trip to Paris about ten years later. They were studying at university and invited me out for a meal in the Latin Quarter, as they knew it was one of my favourite locations. I was amazed to find that they hadn't forgotten the word and agreed that as they were now both adults it was time for me to reveal the meaning. They were genuinely surprised at my answer but saw the funny side of it all. To my horror, I later discovered that there is indeed a ruder definition of the word but I'm not sure whether they ever discovered it.

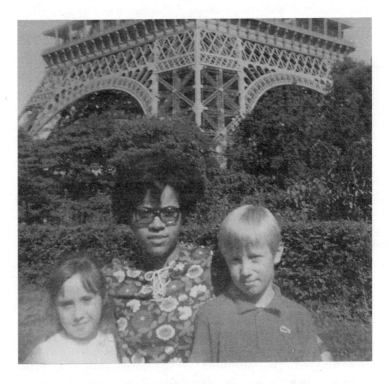

Martine, Jean-Christophe and me, Paris, 1970.

The apartment comprised four bedrooms, two bathrooms, a kitchen and an L-shaped dining room-cum-library. Hanging from ceiling to floor of the library wall was a most beautiful tapestry. There was also a very large balcony that took up two sides of the building and included a small sports area. Everybody made me feel extremely welcome and all occasionally tried to speak some English, with Madame Lacroix being the most proficient. I was asked to consider myself a member of the family and to take all my meals with them. The food was an eye-opener and I was introduced to a wide range of delicious French cuisine! Over and above the fish, steaks, cheese and patisserie, the children insisted I try their snack of a buttered baguette sandwich containing chocolate squares. They were delighted with my very positive reaction. It didn't take me long to become accustomed to strong black coffee, as well as tea with lemon rather than milk.

There was one unfortunate outcome of eating steak tartare. Made from raw ground beef, a raw egg and various seasonings, Madame Lacroix began to get worried when I developed a flu-like illness and swollen glands, so she promptly referred me to a medical specialist in the north of Paris. He seemed to be a very efficient doctor but a man of few words. I'd hardly sat down when he asked me: '*Se pourrait-il que vous soyez enceinte?*' – 'Could you be pregnant?' My immediate thought was, *what the . . . ?* but in spite of my shock, I was able to splutter back, '*Pardon?*' It turned out that he was a specialist in toxoplasmosis, an illness that can cause complications for unborn babies in early pregnancy. The infection, which I did indeed have, can be acquired from cats or eating uncooked meat. There was no treatment given and my symptoms gradually subsided, but the experience put an abrupt halt to eating any more steak tartare.

The need to improve my French was brought home to me pretty quickly when I decided to venture alone into Paris for the first time. The trip entailed taking a bus to reach the nearest metro station. I confidently tried to purchase a ticket from the driver, only for him to start talking to me very quickly. My mind froze, as nothing he said seemed to make any sense. By now a queue of people had formed behind me, and I was feeling very foolish for holding everyone up. Some of them joined in this one-way conversation, making the situation even more incomprehensible. Then a man, speaking some English, explained that for frequent journeys it would be cheaper to buy a book, or carnet, of tickets. So that's what the poor driver had been helpfully trying to tell me.

Prompted by this experience, I registered for French lessons at the Alliance Française in Paris, where I met an American called Sarah, who was in France to study the language. We are still friends, over fifty years later. There were a few initial misunderstandings between us due to our different interpretations of certain words. Two examples come to mind. During a break in the lesson, Sarah asked for directions to the bathroom. 'What?' I responded. 'Don't you have a bath where you live?!' I asked, not realising that she only wanted to find the toilet. Another time she asked me to pass her purse (meaning her whole handbag) and looked askance at me when I started to ferret around inside the handbag looking for it. Fortunately, we both had a good sense of humour.

Sarah recalled some memories from our time in Paris:

We were the only English-speaking students and quickly found each other. We were both young, single and on small budgets! We bonded over croque monsieur or cheap hot dogs for lunch and our almost daily indulgence – French pastries with afternoon tea. You were Elizabeth Furlong then. We talked about everything and anything – the way 22-olds do. You told me about your family, mother and school experiences, particularly an unhappy episode with nuns. Race did not define our relationship – you were Elizabeth, I was Sarah and we were friends.

We enjoyed walking all over the city, visiting museums, going to cheap afternoon movies and talking, talking, talking. The franc was only twenty cents, and therefore five francs to the US dollar. Paris was not horribly expensive *[but I found it was on my initial salary]*; a decent steak/frites dinner might be ten francs – not that we splurged on that very often. We talked about so many things: French history, English history, literature (we both loved to read), English attitudes, American attitudes, French music, the funny differences between American English and English English, crossword puzzles and, of course, boys. Or men, since we were both in our early twenties. We were still so young and carefree and innocent in many ways.

I was a keen photographer and would often go into the city on my own, camera at the ready. To understand what happened next, it is important to remember the context. I arrived in France about eighteen months after the period of rebellion by students and workers that is still referred to as simply Mai Soixante-Huit ('May '68'). The unrest had been particularly intense in the Latin Quarter of Paris where the Sorbonne University is located. Everything was being questioned and challenged, from the education curriculum to the power of the police. Massive demonstrations and strikes had thrown the country into utter turmoil and near collapse. While the iconic President de Gaulle survived the immediate crisis, he was to resign in April 1969 following the rejection of his referendum proposing reform of political institutions.

Sometime in 1970, I decided to take a stroll around the Latin Quarter. There was a small side street lined with police vans (*camions*) that reminded me of the old British Black Marias used to transport prisoners. These *camions* were painted in pale and dark grey, and had criss-cross grilled bars on the two back windows. A police siren light was on the roof. Out came my camera and I took a photo. Suddenly, an armed policeman appeared from nowhere, screamed something at me while lunging at my camera and then tore it away from me. Deaf to my attempts to explain, he was incredibly rude and sneering, telling me that he was taking me to the police station for questioning.

Although initially petrified, a sort of calm came over me as I decided to keep quiet until we arrived. As soon as we went through the doors into the reception, I started to insist very loudly in French that he ring Madame Lacroix at her clinic, stating that she was my 'patron' or boss. His face registered shock at this information and the sudden change in my behaviour. Without argument, he immediately phoned the number and I explained to her what had happened. After she spoke with him, he became very conciliatory and allowed me to leave – with my camera. The photo taken that day is still in my collection. Madame Lacroix was extremely angry about the way I had been treated, going on to tell me about the hostility towards the police in 1968. For my part, I became more vigilant when taking photos, ensuring to keep well away from gendarmes.

Madame Lacroix and I got on extremely well and we loved telling each other funny stories. Very early on during my stay she decided to take me into the city centre for a shopping spree. I squeezed into her little sports car and off we sped on what was to be a quite zany ride. Parking seemed to be impossible near the huge department store of Galeries Lafayette. Then I experienced how it was done! Madame Lacroix bashed her way into an impossibly tiny space. Seeing the fear in my eyes, she told me to relax, as cars had bumpers for a reason! We had such a great time that it was repeated several times during my stay.

The family invited me to spend Christmas 1969 with them. It was a wonderful day, and I was delighted and touched by their great presents – chosen, I think, to encourage my developing enthusiasm for French culture. There was a newly published biography of Edith Piaf written by her half-sister Simone Berteaut. While I knew and loved her songs, it was fantastic to find out more about her – and get to know her repertoire better by listening to the French radio. I also received an LP by the singer Guy Béart, whose sublime voice and lyrics I had already encountered on the radio. I wanted to hear more and went on to buy most of his recordings. His death was announced while I was writing this book, so I took the opportunity to listen to his songs again, now on my iPod.

There were times that I had difficulty in understanding some of the 'argot' or slang words used in Berteaut's book, as they weren't always to be found in my French–English dictionary. One day I made a note of a particular word and asked what it meant at the dinner table. Monsieur Lacroix choked on his food at the other end of the table and his wife tried not to smile, saying it was quite a rude word and she would explain it to me later. It was another salutary lesson – this time to choose a more appropriate time and place to ask questions!

Another book Madame Lacroix bought me was *Papillon* by Henri Charrière, for my birthday in 1970. Published in 1969, it was the autobiography of a prisoner who had escaped from a notorious jail in French Guiana, sparking my curiosity by the immense coverage it received in the media.

The Christmas gift I chose for the children was a record of the musical *Oliver!* that had been such a worldwide hit when the album was released in 1968. Explaining the songs to them provided me with an opportunity to talk about the novels of Charles Dickens. They adored the record and soon learned many of the lyrics.

It didn't take long to discover that most French people take immense pride in their language and can be quite abrupt with anyone who doesn't appear to be trying to learn it. This was certainly the case for Ann, an English nurse I knew who was working at the American Hospital in Paris. She was finding it very difficult to speak French and her stay in the city had turned out so utterly miserable that she was planning to return home (she did stay in the end). For my own part, speaking French as much as possible and not being embarrassed about making mistakes seemed to help, as did not being fazed when corrected sharply by all and sundry.

Nevertheless, speaking mainly French and hearing very little English in those first few months brought on a mild bout of depression. It was a struggle to find the right French words and to speak the language in a grammatically correct manner. I really missed the opportunity of speaking, reading and listening to the English language – later, these experiences gave me some insight into how non-English speaking people must feel when first coming to live in Britain.

It helped to go to the WHSmith bookstore in the Rue

de Rivoli and browse through the newspapers and books, while listening out for people speaking English. I was also a regular visitor to the British Council Library, located in the Rue des Écoles, just off the Boulevard St Michel in the Latin Quarter of Paris. Nesta Roberts was the Paris correspondent for the *Guardian* newspaper, and I learned a great deal from her writings – so much so that I wrote to her, and to my amazement she replied, inviting me to tea at her apartment in Rue de Grenelle in the 6th arrondissement. Her sharp and incisive observations were incredibly refreshing and informative. When she discovered my interest in the events of May 1968, her enthusiastic analysis was probably equivalent to a university tutorial!

My vocabulary gradually expanded through reading French books, and I particularly enjoyed those by Maupassant. The hypocrisy of the French bourgeoisie appears to be a constant theme in his writings, an aspect that I found incredibly entertaining. Françoise Sagan's novel *Bonjour Tristesse* had been a massive hit when published in 1954. It wasn't too difficult to read and it became one of my favourite French novels.

Television programmes were initially very difficult to follow, but I was determined to persevere. An interesting example was the weekly *Les Dossiers de l'Écran*. It featured a film about a topical subject, which I would often find educational and entertaining. There then followed a discussion with a panel of experts that just seemed to go on and on, with everyone shouting over each other. At times it was so frustrating and confusing that I would reluctantly give up and retire to bed with a book. This domineering way of debating appears to continue, judging by current French programmes. Is it a British upbringing that still causes me to find this style of discussion so irritating?

Having said that, I noticed after a while that even this type of debate seemed a little easier to follow. Then came the realisation that I was thinking and counting in French – *et voilà*! The transition had been made, and life started to become so much more bearable and interesting.

But although my French was becoming more fluent, I still wasn't happy with my English accent. Then I read somewhere about the differences in emphasis between syllables spoken in English and French. In the latter it mimics a machine gun, with a very even emphasis given to each syllable, unlike in English. I decided to practise this in my room for the rest of that evening. The next morning, I conversed in this way with the family at breakfast and, to my utter pleasure, was congratulated on not sounding so English.

During the school holidays I would take the children into Paris to wander around the parks and museums or to see a film. One day I took a trip on the metro with Jean-Christophe, Martine and the three-year-old daughter of a French African midwife who worked at the clinic. The little girl began to get very fidgety, so much so that the woman sitting opposite her pulled a face. Unfortunately, the child turned to me and said that the woman was ugly: '*Qu'est-ce qu'elle est moche!*' I immediately reprimanded her and apologised to the woman. She was delighted with my response and said that it was fine and that our children can sometimes embarrass us in public. When I said that the child wasn't my daughter and that London was my home, she complimented me on my French and apologised for her assumption.

My *carte de séjour* or residence permit had been issued in January 1970 and I was thoroughly enjoying my time with the children. The parents provided me with free meals and accommodation, together with a small allowance that was a reasonable amount for the limited amount of work that I was doing. The downside was that the cost of living in France was incredibly expensive. While there was plenty of spare time to explore Paris on my own or with my friend Sarah, I just couldn't afford to. So it was with a heavy heart that after three months, I decided to tell Madame Lacroix of my decision to quit and return to London. She was horrified and sat me down with her husband to discuss an alternative proposition. This was to work nights at the clinic while still continuing to speak English with the children.

As I wasn't a qualified midwife, my areas of work would exclude the labour ward, thank goodness. Rather, I would help the staff to settle the babies and their mothers for the night, and then assist with feeds and breakfasts in the morning. This was ideal, as I adored comforting fretful babies and chatting to the mums, who took great pride in teaching me new French words and correcting my grammar. In the evening, I would feed some of the babies with a sort of pulped carrot juice that sent them soundly off to sleep for the night.

The work offered me the opportunity not only to earn some extra money, but also to practise my French with staff and mothers alike. It was often quiet after midnight, and the staff would let me have a nap for several hours, so it was the best of both worlds. In the morning I would have breakfast with the family upstairs and then usually still have enough energy to set off to Paris to spend time with Sarah. What was even more incredible was that no tax was deducted from my earnings.

Those last six months of my stay were wonderful, as I was very busy and had so much more spending money. Sarah was adept at budgeting and noted all of her daily income and expenditure, a concept alien to me. A few weeks before returning to London I decided to buy a short-wave radio to enable me to continue listening to French radio programmes. To Sarah's horror, I rapidly chose and bought one without checking out other stores for a better bargain. It would take many years before my finances would be managed in a more sensible manner. The radio was fantastic though, providing many hours of listening to those French songs that I had come to love during my stay in Paris.

While working at the clinic I became friends with Paula, a French-Beninese midwife – she was so friendly and feisty, and we got on extremely well. It was Paula who would play such a significant role in enabling me to embrace my Black and African identity and a widening political awareness. It started off during a coffee break, when she asked for my opinion about who was the 'better' colonial power, France or Britain? I honestly hadn't a clue what she was talking about and admitted it.

In response, Paula suggested various books, and the one that had the biggest impact on me was Frantz Fanon's 1952 *Black Skin, White Masks*. Fanon was the first Black author I'd ever read (and, wow, what an author to read); the title says it all. Fanon had practised as a psychiatrist in Algeria and became a political activist in the revolutionary movement for liberation from France. He was to die in 1961 of leukaemia at thirty-six, just three months before Algeria achieved independence.

It was fascinating to explore Fanon's ideas on the psychologically damaging effects of colonialism on Black identity. It abruptly woke me up to the realisation of my own sense of inferiority due to my skin colour. The memories of repeatedly washing my face as a child to become white suddenly came flooding back. It was a relief to discuss it all with Paula, who immediately understood what it was all about and placed it into a broader cultural, political and psychological context; it also made me wonder why I had never properly thought about these issues before.

Thinking about me washing my face in order to be white or my great-aunt saying I was adopted, I had internalised all that shame and stigma as I didn't know anything else. I didn't even have a Black family member – I was the only one in a white family. I'm mixed-race and there are many more mixed-race individuals in the UK nowadays, but they will likely grow up with at least one Black member of their family or have relatives. When you know you're different and you know you stand out, that becomes subliminal. Even the title *Black Skin, White Masks* tells you everything in terms of the psychological harm that is being done to somebody's self-esteem. It will affect people differently – you can have a whole bunch of mixed-race people in a room and their experiences will vary tremendously – but there will be some common themes.

Reading that book, my longstanding negative attitude changed overnight and I decided to stop straightening my hair. I was now imbued with a quiet self-confidence, together with a keen desire to challenge racism whenever possible. There was also a burning need to widen my reading, as I was genuinely horrified at my own ignorance concerning Black culture and politics.

While still enamoured with French culture, I was becoming conscious that their media content was extremely white and Eurocentric. For example, it took many years after leaving Paris before I became aware of the French Caribbean *départements* of Guadeloupe and Martinique, and that the latter was the birthplace of Frantz Fanon. A novel that I should have discovered much earlier is Joseph Zobel's acclaimed autobiographical novel *La Rue Cases-Nègres* (1950, *Black Shack Alley* or *Sugar Cane Alley*). It is set in the 1930s French colony of Martinique and follows the educational success that Zobel achieved, in spite of intense poverty and racism.

During this time, my ambition to become a health visitor never wavered and I made several trips back to London to ensure my place on a course as well as sponsorship from an employing authority. The hovercraft was my favourite form of transport across the English Channel and on one such trip in January 1970, I noticed a Black man staring at me. He eventually approached and apologised for bothering me but wanted to know where I was from. Here we go again, I thought, and trotted out the standard refrain: 'Half-Irish, half-Nigerian and born in Birmingham, England.' He immediately responded: 'But there's no such place as Nigeria, don't you know there's a war on?' The Biafra War had been raging from July 1967 (and would end in the next week or so) and had had huge coverage around the world; the images of pot-bellied starving children had sent out shock waves. While aware of my Nigerian heritage, I had no knowledge of my father, not even his name, and thus felt no personal link to this conflict.

The man continued: 'You look like an Igbo, it's really important that you find out about your father.' It was so interesting to hear him talk about the war and about the plight of the Igbo people. Many years later, I was to read of a similar encounter experienced by Jackie Kay, the Scottish-Nigerian poet and novelist who had been adopted from birth. In *Red Dust Road*, her 2010 memoirs of tracing both biological parents, she describes how a man she met on a train in Manchester told her that she looked Igbo. It was to prove correct for both of us. The hovercraft encounter, together with my greater interest in Black history, made me start thinking about my dad.

Chapter 24:

A Radical Health Visitor

The young woman who returned to London in the summer of 1970 was very different from the one who left nine months before. Now fluent in French, I was more mature and self-confident and much happier. I felt more at ease with both my white Irish and Black Nigerian heritage and I was keen to become involved in Black community activities. I was also starting my health visitor's course at Chiswick Polytechnic. The London Borough of Brent had sponsored my place and would be providing me with employment once I qualified. The one-year programme was a combination of college-based lectures and observation visits, followed by a two-month supervised placement at a child health clinic in Wembley, Brent.

I also needed to find accommodation urgently. Fortunately, it wasn't that difficult and I was soon sharing a flat just off the high street in Acton with Pippa, a student teacher. It was to prove a great success, as we hit it off straightaway, thankfully. We were both very engaged in politics and signed up to the local Labour Party together. I would happily spend time at home watching TV, knitting and listening to music and I got on well with Pippa's boyfriend, who would visit her.

Life outside studies was now much more attractive than it had been and while I enjoyed some of the lectures, others were somewhat tedious. (On returning there years later to give a talk on sickle cell disease, a former tutor informed the class that a public health doctor had complained to her once that I was doing a crossword puzzle during his lecture. That particular session must have been incredibly boring, as it was one of my favourite subjects.)

The principal tutor was a far cry from Miss Papa of my student nursing days. I found her very po-faced and was frustrated that she wouldn't call on me when I put my hand up. She seemed taken aback that I'd go to the House of Commons to listen to debates and talk about current affairs and recent legislation in tutorials. I was articulate and asked a lot of questions and I got the impression she wasn't happy that I was so political. Let's just say that I wasn't one of her favourite students, although I was never quite sure why. So it was extremely enlightening to receive this recollection by Sue, a fellow student at the time: 'My lasting memory of you is of a feisty and questioning fellow student – displaying extreme tolerance of that awful principal tutor and her racially discriminating attitude towards you!'

I found being on placement at the child health clinic so much more interesting than the lectures, as it included visiting families in their homes, predominantly focusing on mothers and their young children. The community was very diverse, comprising mainly white British, Irish, Caribbean and South Asian families. Many of the latter had fled Uganda and Kenya after their independence from Britain in 1962 and 1963 respectively. Faced with surrendering their British passports for Kenyan citizenship, 50,000 Asian Kenyans had migrated to Britain but were unable to bring their wealth with them, so faced terrible living and working conditions.[1] Alarmed by the number of migrants, the British government also tightened immigration controls in 1968, demanding Asian Kenyans had work permits or close relatives living in the country.[2]

Similarly, after Uganda's independence, its leader Idi Amin (a despot known as the Butcher of Uganda) accused the country's Asian minority (who had been encouraged to settle there by the British administration as a buffer between Europeans and Africans in the middle rungs of commerce and administration) of disloyalty and non-integration, calling them 'bloodsuckers'. In August 1972, they were given ninety days to leave the country or face being imprisoned in military camps – and around 27,200 emigrated to the UK.[3] Facing a mixed reception from the British government, which initially tried to place the migrants on islands such as the Falklands, the arrival of Asian Ugandans has since been described as 'one of the most successful moments in UK immigration history' and provided a major boost to the country's economy (it's estimated the migrant community created 30,000 jobs in Leicester alone).[4]

As these families tried to find support in Britain, it took a few years for a Gujarati-speaking health visitor to be appointed and to signpost them to local health services. I was to learn a great deal from her about people's cultural beliefs in respect to nutrition, childbirth and parenting. She would explain eating habits – types of meat or vegetarianism – the different branches of Hinduism or traditions around the baby (one day I found a coin under a baby's head and their mother explained it was one of their traditions). She was also really good at explaining the political situation in East Africa – what these families had been through and why they had certain outlooks.

I still have a small red diary for 1971 in which for some unknown reason I decided to record brief notes concerning daily activities and occasional observations. This was the only year I documented my life in such detail. It's turned out to be a very useful record and something of an eye-opener. Some of the comments now seem naive and occasionally downright crass, but most are helpful recollections of my life and views as a 24-year-old. Without it, there is no way I could have recalled the minutiae of what had clearly been an incredibly hectic period.

The diary revealed I had an unhealthy start to 1971 due to becoming ill with bronchitis and asthma. The end of the year was no better, apparently, as my mother comments in a letter to me in early 1972: 'I hope you are keeping well and not overdoing it. You didn't seem at all well at Christmas. Look after yourself.' There is a brief entry about spending a few days in Wolverhampton at Christmas. I can't remember any details, but by now I was in more regular contact with my mother and this holiday visit was a rare overnight stay. A month later, ten-year-old Pam wrote a sweet letter thanking me for the very popular present of a record player. She added that it helped cut down the amount of time they were now watching telly and 'it stops Mum putting so much money into the TV slot meter'.

Apart from college lectures, the months that followed were occupied with going to hear a host of speakers at meetings arranged by the Fabian Society, Labour Party, Socialist Medical Association (SMA) and the more radical Needle health group. The latter was my favourite organisation, and I was involved with it for a couple of years. The name came from the title of a magazine they produced, the purpose of which was to well and truly 'needle' those trying to dismantle the NHS. Members were drawn from all sectors of the health service and included nurses, students, technicians, porters and doctors. Needle challenged, among other issues, the growth of private practice within the NHS, nursing culture, inadequate mental health services and reorganisation of the NHS.

(Although I am unable to recall meeting her then, it turned out that one of the medical students had been Dr Moira Dick. She was also a member of the SMA. I came to know Moira well in the 1980s through our mutual work on sickle cell disease, when she was a consultant community child health specialist in south London. It was only after we had both retired that these common links became apparent. As well as that, she had studied at Newnham College, Cambridge. What a small world.)

Through attending these various meetings, I was able to listen to Martin Ennals, human rights activist and Secretary General of Amnesty. Other speakers included Labour politicians such as Ennals' brother David, Harold Wilson, Barbara Castle, Richard Crossman and Dr John Dunwoody. There were also talks by newspaper editors such as the *Guardian's* Alastair Hetherington and William Rees-Mogg of *The Times*.

By now my pride and joy was a wonderful orange Mobylette scooter, purchased through monthly payments. It was in France that I first appreciated their incredible popularity, as they were such an inexpensive form of transport. The Mobylette offered me a brilliant and cheap way of zipping around London (and going to France for a summer holiday) as the fuel consumption was very efficient, although it was prone to breakdowns. One day, I took my friend Helen (sitting on the passenger seat) on a trip to Hyde Park Corner. When we prepared to leave, the scooter wouldn't start and I had to push it five miles back to Acton. The only comment in my diary is 'Exhausted'. It took nearly a week to repair the damage, which had been caused by somebody putting half a pound of sugar in the fuel tank. A year on, when a motorist ignored my right of way and crashed into me, I reluctantly decided to think about saving to buy a second-hand car.

Unsurprisingly during this phase of my life, many of the books I read were political in nature. One that had a great impact was the fantastic and searing *The Ragged Trousered Philanthropists*, the 1914 novel by Robert Tressell. It really brought poor, working-class existence to life in the way that Dickens's books can.

My diary entry for Sunday, 21 February records: 'Woke at 10 a.m., bright cold day. Went to Trafalgar Square to watch TUC demonstration, had a good view – sunny day. Watched TV & finished book.' Searching the internet helped me to discover that over 200,000 people had marched that day from Hyde Park to Trafalgar Square, protesting against the proposed Industrial Relations Act.

During the Easter holidays of 1971, I flew to stay with a friend in Dublin. On a hot Easter Sunday we visited Phoenix Park, followed the next day by a trip to Glendale. We also visited Avoca in County Wicklow, an incredibly beautiful town. The following Tuesday, we hitch-hiked up to Belfast to start our travels around Northern Ireland, staying at youth hostels and once with a friend's relative.

Our itinerary included Belfast, Downings in County Donegal, then Portrush and along the stunning North Antrim coast, taking in the magnificent Giant's Causeway. This was three years after the start of the Troubles. We were to learn the opposing points of view as we obtained lifts from both Protestants and Catholics. One of the latter told us proudly that he had nine children and that there would be more in order to ensure that the Protestants didn't wipe them out. A Protestant driver addressed our ignorance concerning William of Orange with a history lesson about the Battle of the Boyne. As we had reached our destination before it was finished, he just pulled over and continued for about fifteen minutes.

Young and innocent, we had little sense of fear throughout the journey, although quite conscious of the ongoing conflict. While aware of my family links with Wexford, I later discovered that my grandmother's family originated from Moygannon, as well as Rostrevor and Warrenpoint in County Down. They became part of Northern Ireland following the partition of the country in 1921.

Back in London, I was becoming more involved with the local Labour Party and became Assistant Secretary, then Treasurer. My diary records canvassing with my flatmate for the May 1971 local elections and that Labour gained a majority of seats on the council. While interested in listening to visiting speakers and attending demonstrations, there was a more tedious side to some of the meetings. An observation I made about the Annual General Meeting was: 'usual stifling petty arrangements'. There were also very few, if any, discussions concerning minority and immigrant communities, and I was conscious of being the only Black member at meetings. I decided to become more involved with the Black community and meet more Black people, and started to hear about meetings via flyers and word of mouth.

As a result, in June 1971 I volunteered to do Saturday work for the Ealing Community Relations Council and helped out at various school projects. The first one was held at the Dominion Cinema in Southall, where helpers taught forty children. On Saturday, 9 October I became involved with one in Acton: '1st day of Saturday school. 64 children arrived. Bit chaotic but worthwhile.' The following week, sixty-five turned up and it was more organised and settled. That same evening, I went to Ealing Town Hall for the Caribbean Overseas Association (COA) anniversary dance, where a steel band played. A few months earlier, the COA hall had been set on fire and I noted that this was now the third arson attack: 'wrecking hope of having a project there. Wrote letter to *Acton Gazette*.' I can't recall if it was ever published.

It was through these projects that I became acquainted with Jessica Huntley and her fellow Guyanese husband, Eric.[5] The couple had set up the UK's second Black publishing company, Bogle L'Ouverture Publications – named after the freedom fighters Paul Bogle (from Jamaica) and Toussaint L'Ouverture (from Haiti). They published writers including the Guyanese radical historian Walter Rodney and Lucy Safo (whose 1993 book, *Cry a Whisper*, went on to win the Commonwealth Writers' Prize for Best First Book) and poetry by Lemn Sissay and Valerie Bloom. (John La Rose and his partner, Sarah White, had also set up New Beacon Books in 1966, and they were friends with Jessica and Eric; both wanted to address the paucity of Black writing in mainstream publishing.)

Since arriving in London during the late 1950s, Jessica and Eric had become known for their pioneering Black politics and activism and were responsible for founding the Caribbean Education and Community Workers Association (CECWA), the first specialist Black education group to have been established in the UK, and the Black Parents Movement (BPM), among many others. They also helped to organise the 1981 Black People's Day of Action march that attracted 20,000 Black Britons from all over the country and was the largest protest march of its kind at the time. It followed the deaths of thirteen young Black people during a house fire at a party in New Cross and the consequent outrage at the failure of authorities to take any serious interest in the tragedy – hence the slogan 'Thirteen dead and nothing said'.

In 1974, they opened The Bookshop in West Ealing, but before then I would help to sell their books at community events all over London and – when I had a car – further afield in places such as the St Paul's Festival (now Carnival) in Bristol. Basically, at any event where there could be a bookstall at the back of the hall.

While Eric and Jessica worked together, for me, Jessica was the dominant force. She frightened the life out of me when I first met her because she would say what she wanted to say whether you liked it or not. I admired her and loved what she was doing with the books and their strong Black network. At this point, I was footloose and fancy-free, and Jessica soon realised I could be a useful volunteer because I had a lovely little second-hand cream Mini. Jessica didn't really ask you; she told you. Initially, I didn't stand up to her, but once I got through her wall of assertiveness, I discovered she had a lovely sense of humour, and she became a very good friend and educator to me. She was very kind, open and enabling, and she was very proud of me as she hadn't come across many Black health radicals.

We both learned and gained from each other, and this was really when my Black history education began. Sitting behind the Bogle-L'Ouverture Publications bookstall before events kicked off or during a boring session, it gave me a chance to pick up a book and read. Books such as *The Lonely Londoners* (1956) by Trinidadian author Samuel Selvon, Eldridge Cleaver's 1968 memoir *Soul on Ice* and the 1971 edition of Paul Robeson's *Here I Stand*. I also read Walter

Rodney's seminal *How Europe Underdeveloped Africa* (1972), which outlines how European imperialists exploited then neglected the development of the continent.

When it was released, the book was hailed in Tanzania as 'probably the greatest book event in Africa since Frantz Fanon'.[6] As Rodney's publisher, Jessica asked me to drive him to various meetings during his visits to London from Tanzania and then Guyana. We were to become firm friends. A tiny, tiny guy, he was so bright, an incredible intellectual, a brilliant orator and he also had a great sense of humour; we'd have long conversations as we drove around. Rodney would tell me about who he was meeting and where he was going to speak.

He was like the Caribbean Nelson Mandela, because he was a courageous individual who put his head above the parapet working for racial justice and equality across the globe. He was feared by governments because he was so bright and because of the influence he had in different sections of the community, from Black people to students. He was such a pleasant guy with a lovely grin, but if anyone tried to argue with him, he'd be able to reach for facts and you just couldn't get one past him. He was a Pan-Africanist, so not just looking at our situation as a Black individual in our own area but how it fit in with a post-colonial world – how did it fit in with people in the Caribbean or Africa? A lot of his work was in Tanzania, and he was expelled from Jamaica because he was thought to be too radical; this led to the 1968 Rodney riots.

It was around this time I also read Nelson Mandela's 'I Am Prepared to Die' speech at the start of the Rivonia Trial in 1964, which had a huge impact on me, and *Angela Davis: An Autobiography* (1974). It was thrilling to hear her speak at the London Keskidee Centre on 10 December 1974, and I still have the black and white photos that I took of her at this event. She brought to life the issues surrounding racism in the US, such as police brutality (and we're now reliving so many of these moments). She also brought the Black woman's perspective, and she was such an international figure that I loved her and was very drawn to her. There was a huge campaign to free her when she was imprisoned; you catch your breath and hope these people are going to survive, and she did.

Looking back, I was so fortunate to be part of this time because it moulded my belief system and introduced me to a wonderful set of people, some of whom I'm still in contact with. It gave me the confidence to counter experiences of racism and to deal with it while not being overwhelmed. It influenced how I brought up my daughter and her values. Looking at everything we're going through now – in this era of Black Lives Matter – you realise it's continuous. And how do different people deal with it? How do the media deal with it? Some of the excuses given and how repetitive they are . . . But also what cheers you up is the support that you see and the fact that people are being educated in terms of what's going on.

Getting involved with Jessica, reading Black literature, listening to Black speakers and going to cultural events (after all, it wasn't all politics), I was mixing much more with Black people. There were hardly any television programmes and there was no internet at the time. Yes, there were books by Black writers, but if those books aren't recommended to you at school or available in the library, how are you going to know about them? We're all brought up in bubbles – Black, white, women, men – it takes other people or experiences to make you realise what goes on elsewhere. Embracing my Black culture was both cathartic and exhilarating; it brought me joy and changed the way I saw the world.

Chapter 25:

Speaking Out

Having finished the written health visitor exams, I started a two-month period of supervised health visiting practice in Wembley as part of my training. It was a happy and interesting experience, as it involved a very small caseload of families with young children, which fitted my interests perfectly. All was going well until I spotted an anomaly in the way that one section of the weekly statistics were being completed.

Health visitors were asked to record the number of families they had seen who were from the 'New Commonwealth'. When I asked the first health visitor for the definition of this term, she was quite upfront and said she wasn't sure but thought it was non-white families. The next one replied: 'Well, people like you, dear.' This patronising comment galvanised me into questioning as many other health visitors as possible. Their answers included 'Black people', 'Indians', 'non-English speakers' and 'recent immigrants'.

Me: 'From any country?'

Reply: 'Er, no, just countries like Africa.'

Me: 'That's a continent.'

[Silence.]

Finally, this intriguing one: 'You know, people with funny names.'

The New Commonwealth was a term referring primarily to recently decolonised and predominantly non-white countries in the Caribbean, Africa and South Asia. I explored the reason for collecting these statistics and discovered that it was in order to claim Section 11 funds. These were available from the Local Authority for the provision of services specifically relevant for immigrant communities. So this led me to investigate if any funding had been obtained, as I'd observed there weren't any interpreters to assist health visitors, which would have been very helpful. This line of questioning was a step too far for my health visitor supervisor. Despite her previous glowing reports, she determined that my attitude wasn't conducive to health visiting and proceeded to fail my practice assessment. This meant that I wouldn't be able to become a health visitor.

I was so angry. One aspect of my developing self-esteem was that I knew I was intelligent and had passed all the theoretical exams without any difficulties. Therefore, the background of why I had been failed was so unjust. There was no logical reason for it happening. Fortunately, my contacts with Needle meant I approached a member of the Socialist Medical Association, who advised that I speak to Dr Ernest Grundy, the local medical officer of health. What a breath of fresh air it was to meet up with him. First off, he actually congratulated me on my actions, then immediately ordered a review of how the New Commonwealth statistics were being collated and how any funding was being used. Representations were also made to the college about the threat to fail me. I was called to appear before a panel to confirm my final results. My diary records on Friday, 22 August that I sat outside room 222 for one hour before being informed that 'there would be no necessity for me to see the examiners'. The next day a letter arrived confirming my status as a qualified health visitor.

Thinking about what I experienced makes me realise that this discrimination can still happen, and I ask myself, are those examples hidden or not? Is it easier to deal with now? I often share this experience in my talks in case people think, *oh, it'll never happen to me.* In my situation, it was down to a broader aspect of racism. When you're cocooned from it, it's a big shock when it happens to you.

Now that I had my qualification, I started work as a health visitor in September 1971. My base was a small child health clinic located in the grounds of One Tree Hill park in the Alperton district of Wembley. At this time, community child health services were managed by the local authority (their transfer to the NHS took place in 1974). Miss Sansom was the only other health visitor there, a much older and very experienced practitioner whom I liked and greatly respected. She was happy to advise me in those early days, then allowed me the freedom to innovate where I saw fit. This included collaborating with a male social worker to set up a mother and toddler group that for the first eight months met on a weekly basis in the clinic. When the numbers regularly reached twenty to thirty, it moved to larger premises in a local youth and community centre, courtesy of the education department.

The group was established after I'd observed that many mothers came to the clinic every single week to weigh their healthy, thriving babies. One day, there was an incredibly long queue and I apologised for the delay but also asked why they came so often. The response of one mother, 'To get out of the house and have a chat with an adult!' was greeted with nods and a round of applause. The successful outcome of the group in reducing their feelings of isolation was written up in my first-ever published article in the now defunct *Nursing Mirror & Midwives Journal* and was entitled 'A Mothers' Group in Alperton' in 1975. On rereading it so many years later, I noted that while Asian and Caribbean mothers attended, they were few in number, which was probably due to the isolation of minority ethnic groups in our communities, and that – due to lack of experience – a group like this might make them anxious or wary. Also, I don't know if they would even have heard about it. One can't assume . . .

It was so liberating to make links with a wide variety of people who could help to solve problems encountered by families. For example, a local councillor was quick to resolve one for a family with three small children. Visiting them during a particularly cold spell, I discovered the mother and toddlers huddled around an open oven in the kitchen. They had no heating in their council house and were just being passed from pillar to post by various officials. The councillor and I were to become close colleagues and he often expressed a wish that more professionals would contact him about issues in his local ward.

I made it a priority to visit the general practice that many families were registered with and was fortunate to meet Dr Walker, the senior partner, and Megan, the practice nurse. She recalled:

> You came as our new health visitor in 1971 and were very different from any previous ones we had ever had. You weren't just interested in health; it was also the much broader aspects of people. This was because the area that you were working in had quite a lot of social and financial problems. You certainly would come back and

discuss with Dr Walker and put people in touch with the right people to make sure they were getting the correct benefits. This may well have been your role, but I can't ever remember any other health visitor talking about that sort of thing before. So I was very conscious of the fact that you connected with people on a different level. You were concerned about them and you wanted to help them. It wasn't just going to see the baby, which people often thought that's what a health visitor did – no, it was far broader. I remember you being happy and confident.

This last sentence is striking, as Megan was the first person to describe me as being confident. It is a sharp contrast to that shy student nurse in Paddington and can be attributed not only to maturity, but also to a growing inner sense of self-worth, gained from my wider experience of life and increasing radicalisation. Megan continued: 'You've never been a pushover at all; you've always had a strong sense of justice and you feel strongly about things that you consider right.'

There were three families on my caseload that had children with genetic blood conditions. The first had a boy and a girl who were non-identical twins, whom I visited frequently from birth. Their mother was very anxious, as they were her first and only children, and the initial problems were typical queries relating to feeding and sleeping patterns. She was also very isolated and, at times, tired and depressed. As the twins got older, I would see them peering out of the window and becoming more excited as I walked down the path to their front door. They were a delightful pair.

One seemed to be underweight and pale, so I asked Dr Walker for his advice. He asked to see the two of them and, to everybody's shock, blood tests revealed that both had thalassaemia major. This is an inherited anaemia due to inadequate haemoglobin production and requires lifelong blood transfusions. At this time in the UK, the condition was mainly seen in Greek and Turkish Cypriots and South Asian communities. One reason for our surprise was that one of the parents was white English, although I later learned that the latter have a 1 in 1000 chance of being a healthy thalassaemia carrier.[1]

Two other children on my patch had sickle cell anaemia – an inherited anaemia that causes severe, painful crises. One of the mothers had gone to the public library to find out more, only to be devastated on reading that it was a disease 'that affected Negro children who rarely survive beyond two years of age'. This information was grossly out of date in both prognosis and in the use of the word 'Negro'. At that time, I didn't know anything about either thalassaemia or sickle cell disease and I couldn't have predicted that I would specialise in both and reconnect with these children into their adulthood. This revealed my appalling ignorance about it (we'd never been taught about it) and my inability to be of much help to the devastated parents.

As I researched it further, I would learn that sickle cell disease is an inherited anaemia affecting the haemoglobin inside the red blood cells. It originated in those parts of the tropics where falciparum malaria is prevalent – and children under two years with sickle cell trait have partial protection against the worst effects of this severe malaria. Sickle cell trait is found in one in four Nigerians and one in ten of the African-Caribbean population. It also affects other groups in the UK with origins in South Asia, the Mediterranean and the Middle East – so it has an impact on a wide range of people (and is not confined to members of the Black community, as many still believe). Blue-eyed, fair-haired, white individuals can also inherit the condition or the trait.[2]

Sickle cell trait, or the carrier state, can be detected by a simple and cheap blood test at any time during a person's life. Although they might not have the illness, if they have a child with someone who also has the trait, there is a 25 per cent chance that each of their children will inherit sickle cell disease. There is also a 75 per cent chance that each child is healthy, either through inheriting sickle cell trait (50 per cent chance) or the usual haemoglobin type (25 per cent chance).

There are several types of sickle cell disease, the most common being sickle cell anaemia (Hb SS), while the others are sickle beta^0 thalassaemia (which is usually as severe as Hb SS), Hb SC disease and sickle beta^0 thalassaemia. These latter two are generally milder, but this is not always the case. Sickling of the red blood cells can cause them to change shape to one resembling a farmer's sickle or a banana. This then blocks the flow of blood, creating mild to life-threatening complications.[3]

The condition can be extremely varied and very unpredictable. Painful crises are the most common problem. They can be mild or so excruciating that hospital admission is required for treatment with drugs such as morphine. Severe infections are common, requiring a daily preventative dose of antibiotics during early childhood. Complications of sickling can affect many parts of the body such as the lungs, kidneys, eyes, hips and shoulders. It can also cause strokes from childhood onwards. While survival is improving, the illness can still result in early deaths. US authors Claster and Vichinsky noted in a November 2003 *British Medical Journal* article that the average lifespan of seventeen years in 1973 had, three decades later, increased to fifty.

The NHS National Haemoglobinopathy Registry Annual Data Report for 2019/2020 records a total of 12,659 sickle cell patients. In comparison, the Cystic Fibrosis (CF) Trust states that there are over 10,000 people with CF, an inherited illness affecting the lungs and digestive system. CF mainly affects white Northern Europeans and, less frequently, Black and minority ethnic groups. The NHS Screening Programme in England for 2017–2018 reported 262 babies screening positive for Cystic Fibrosis and 252 for sickle cell disease.[4]

From the early 1980s, it has become possible to detect whether an unborn baby has sickle cell anaemia, although the testing procedure carries a risk of miscarriage. The couple then has to make the complex decision of whether to terminate or to continue the pregnancy. Meeting these families was one of the first triggers that led to sickle cell disease becoming so crucial to my career later on.[5]

Chapter 26:

Breaking Out

On 11 September 1971, a few weeks after qualifying as a health visitor, I embarked on my first trip to the US. It was organised at a very affordable price by the Fabian Society in partnership with Americans for Democratic Action (ADA). Our three-week programme of activities commenced in New York before moving on to Philadelphia and ending in Washington DC. Ann Clwyd MP (then Ann Roberts, working as a journalist) was one of the members of the group and we were to become friends. (In fact, Ann was the only member from the British group with whom I would continue to keep in touch. She'd later invite me for wonderful visits to Cardiff, where I met her journalist husband, Owen, who later became Head of Programmes at BBC Wales. One memorable trip included several days on the beautiful Gower Peninsula. Owen was an erudite and gentle person who was later diagnosed with multiple sclerosis. It was devastating to hear Ann speak in Parliament about the poor care he received at the time of his death in 2012.)

In 1971, Ann was on the Welsh Hospital Board as a lay member. The board ran the whole of the health service in Wales until the Tories abolished it in 1974, transferring its responsibilities to the Welsh Office. She recalled of the trip: 'We were with a group of people who had a particular interest in the health service, do you remember? We started talking and sort of palled up together. You came over as a very caring person, very determined, you asked questions that some people might not ask, you weren't afraid to ask them. I just saw you as a sort of fellow spirit, actually.'

Then she described an incident that I had completely forgotten:

I remember on our first stop in New York, we were sitting on high stools in the breakfast room and this porter just fell. You thought he might have had a heart attack and, as a nurse, you immediately went over to him. I remember the scene very well and you tried to loosen his tie and they said, 'Stop, don't touch him.' I remember how surprised we all were! 'You've got to first check his medical insurance status.' They decided which ambulance to call. That gave me a shock and I'm sure it certainly gave you one, as well.

That was our introduction to the US health service.

Ann remembered that a lot of people wanted to meet us to learn more about the NHS. 'This was particularly the case for those who were then prominent in the Democratic Party, so we met people like Hubert Humphrey and the Kennedys.' Our meeting with Senator Ted Kennedy in Washington DC remains a vivid memory, as he came bouncing up to us with a huge grin on his face and gave me a very firm handshake. Smiling and ebullient, he plied us with his searching questions about health visiting and community health services.

It was a volatile time to be in the US. During a sightseeing trip to New York's Times Square on 13 September 1971, I happened to look up at the zipper (a moving illuminated bulletin board). It was showing news of the deaths of ten hostages and twenty-nine inmates following the storming of Attica Prison by state troopers. Governor Nelson Rockefeller had given the order after a four-day occupation following a riot about prison conditions and the murder of a prison guard.

There was also a lot of tension between the police and the radical organisation the Black Panthers. In 1969, then director of the FBI J. Edgar Hoover described the party as 'the greatest threat to the internal security of the country' and, in 1970, imprisoned founder Bobby Seale was charged with ordering the killing of police informant Alex Rackley.[1] Before leaving London, I'd been given the address of a New York Chapter of the Black Panther Party, somewhere off Harlem's 125th Street, and I was determined to visit. I asked a man for directions and, once he realised I was from England, he said he'd take me there as it wasn't advisable to wander around on my own in the area. On our arrival, someone peered through a grill asking for the name that my London contact had given me then unlocked the door.

I was escorted downstairs to a small basement room, where a group of about fourteen youths were huddled together taking turns to read aloud from a book. This turned out to be *Soledad Brother: The Prison Letters of George Jackson*, published in 1970. Silently, they shuffled up to make a space to sit, then I waited somewhat nervously for the book to reach me. When I began to read, there were shocked faces and shouts of incredulity. 'You from England, sister?!' The book was taken from me and friendly questions were fired left, right and centre. When the session ended and it transpired that I was on my own, a couple of them were charged with accompanying me back to the subway. It was an exhilarating meeting and was one of the most incredible and heart-warming experiences of my stay.

Another unforgettable event in New York was when our British delegation met Bayard Rustin, the noted African-American civil rights and gay activist. He was the organiser of the 1963 March on Washington for Jobs and Freedom, attended by over 200,000 people and led by Revd Martin Luther King Jr and others.[2] I was enthralled by his succinct and vivid accounts of key moments in the history of the civil rights movement. He also provided background information about the Attica Prison situation. So, it was with utter horror and embarrassment to hear one of our group smugly state that Britain didn't have any similar incidents. Quick as a flash and in his impeccable way of speaking, Rustin retorted sarcastically: 'Didn't you all have something called the Notting Hill riots in 1958?' (This had been violent riots between white Teddy boys in London and counterattacks from the Black Caribbean population.)[3]

When the meeting ended, one of the organisers handed me a note from Rustin asking me to come and have a chat with him. At this period, I had a huge afro and during the trip was often mistaken for an African-American. As soon as I said a few words, Rustin burst out laughing and said he had been wondering why I was with the group. We discussed the nature and objectives of the trip in more detail. He asked me whether I would like to learn more about civil rights during my stay in Washington DC and, of course, the answer was a resounding yes.

To my astonishment, Rustin asked me to accompany him to a room where there was a phone, took out his bulging address book and proceeded to call several people. They were informed about my visit and asked to brief me on their history as well as show me around various projects and organisations. One such person was Marion Barry, who would be elected eight years later for the first of four terms of office as mayor of Washington DC. Back in that autumn of 1971, Marion took me on a conducted tour of an organisation he had co-founded called Pride Inc. It offered an opportunity for jobless Black youths to work their way up the employment ladder. This started with rat catching and cleaning streets, with the possibility of progressing to leadership roles in fuel stations owned by Pride.

There's no doubt that I returned to London a changed and more informed person. In the autumn of 1972, my local Labour branch chose me as a delegate to attend the Annual Party Conference being held in Blackpool. Ann was also going and invited me to share a flat she was renting for the week. As a result of her contacts and introductions, I was able to observe at close quarters key players within the Labour Party. While it made for an incredibly interesting week, it was here that it dawned on me that I wasn't cut out to be a Labour Party activist, as I was growing increasingly disillusioned with it.

In Ealing, a few members were privately raising concerns about discriminatory behaviour towards Asians attempting to join a particular Labour-run social club. I was unimpressed by the apathetic responses that led to no action at the time; it reminded me of the notorious colour bar in 1964 at a Labour club in the West Midlands town of Smethwick. This was the year that Labour, led by Harold Wilson, won the general election, but Smethwick bucked the trend and voted in Peter Griffiths, a right-wing Conservative candidate associated with the slogan: 'If you want a nigger for a neighbour, vote Labour.' (Two years later, the actor Andrew Faulds regained the seat for Labour.)

While I was appreciative of many of the Labour Party priorities, it became clear to me that I was living in two worlds. There were so many problems affecting minority communities that were barely being addressed; one example was the bussing of Black and minority ethnic pupils in Southall to schools outside the area. A policy was in place where the number of Black and minority ethnic pupils could not exceed 30 per cent in any one school and had begun in Ealing in 1963, due to the concerns of white parents. It would result in the murder of Shakil Malik in 1974, who was bottled to death when boarding his school bus. Following the prosecution of Ealing Local Education Authority in 1975, bussing on the grounds of ethnicity alone was ruled discriminatory under the 1968 Race Relations Act.[4]

Looking back, I had wanted to get involved with politics and I had done it in an Establishment-traditional way. But I then realised: my goodness – this is ethnocentric. They're not even addressing issues on their doorstep, or when the odd member does want to address things, they don't get the support. I eventually decided not to renew my membership.

Then, in 1972, I met Peter Moses, another friend of the publisher Jessica Huntley, who was a gentle, intelligent and wonderful guy and very passionate about Black activism. Peter was also one of the pioneers behind the Marcus Garvey Saturday Supplementary School in Hammersmith, which was run by parents, teachers and volunteers. It had been created as a way to provide a place for Black children to learn about their culture and history, but was also partly a response to Bernard Coard's 1971 book *How the West Indian Child Is Made Educationally Sub-normal in the British School System: The Scandal of the Black Child in Schools in Britain*, which was published by New Beacon Books. In it, Coard outlined how the British school system was disproportionately and wrongly removing Black children (especially from the British African-Caribbean community) from mainstream education and placing them in educationally subnormal (ESN) schools (which had previously been labelled 'schools for the mentally subnormal'), affecting both their education and economic prospects.

Peter invited me and a group of like-minded Black volunteers to help out at the Saturday School that he'd co-founded with Dada Imarogbe, a fellow Dominican. The school was held in the afternoons in a small basement off the Uxbridge Road. I was to work there for more than two years with a group of enthusiastic activists, some of whom are still my friends to this day. The project was self-organised and located in a cold basement kept warm by paraffin heaters.

Over forty years later, six of them met up with me to record our memories of those heady times. As well as Dada, they included Marvlyn, Sandra, Florence, Rose and Mariamma. We recalled trips made with the children to places they had never been – Brighton comes to mind, and the Tutankhamun exhibition at the British Museum. One of our charges was the future film-maker and artist Steve McQueen, who for a brief period came to the school with his sister when he was very young. In 2020, he made the film *Education* as part of his BBC Small Axe anthology, which was inspired by Coard's book and his own experiences of ESN schools. He later told the *Guardian* that the Saturday School fostered '[his] love of art' which 'opened [his] world'.[5]

My friends remember me variously as 'always questioning, wanting to know everything', 'an eager beaver', 'into textbooks' and 'prepared to put the effort in'. As far as my being mixed-race was concerned, none of them seem to have thought about it. Most just assumed that, like them, I would have a Caribbean or West African heritage, remembering me as friendly and with a big smile, noting my big hair, that I came 'from somewhere up north' and even that I was 'very posh'! It was wonderful to chat in this way and the surprise was how so many memories came flooding back. The group was probably unaware of the influential role they played in assisting me to absorb so much about Black British history and culture. This was a period of transition from a virtually all-white environment to that of a more ethnically diverse one.

Peter sadly died of leukaemia on 20 December 1972, at just twenty-seven years of age. His death occurred only months after he had fulfilled his dream of setting up the Saturday School. Peter had also been very active in raising funds for other projects, such as the first ever Black Arts Festival in 1972. It was held at St Thomas Hall in Shepherd's Bush and my diary records that I attended the event on Sunday, 28 May. This was the same venue where hundreds of us would gather the following year at a cultural memorial concert to celebrate Peter's life and honour this charismatic and committed activist. Unfortunately, many incorrectly perceived he'd died of sickle cell anaemia, so I tried to explain the difference between it and leukaemia, only to realise I only knew more about the latter disease thanks to my nursing education. It was then that Jessica Huntley challenged my own lack of knowledge: 'If you as a Black nurse don't know about this, then how are we meant to?' It was a question that would stay with me.

Throughout this time, the thought of finding my father had been sitting at the back of my mind. It was building and building, and I realised I needed to get the full picture. Even though I'd been brought up in a totally white environment and acted as a 'white English' person (because I didn't have any other influences), society kept reminding me I was brown. From the washing of my face and the constant questions like: 'Where are you from? No, where are you *really* from?' Then to me gradually realising that the colour of my skin was different from everybody else's and wondering, *why isn't anyone in my family talking about it?* – the very fact no one had even spoken about my father was a big signal that this wasn't something to be acknowledged.

It was such a huge stigma, from my mum being an unmarried mother to my father being Black. I used to have questions running through my mind such as: *what might I find? Should I even go along this path? And how will I even do it?* But now things had changed, I had transitioned to: *there's nothing wrong with being brown-skinned – come on, Elizabeth – find your father.* So in March 1972, I at last wrote to my mother asking her for the name and any other details concerning my Nigerian father – asking via letter meant I could lessen the impact of the question.

Chapter 27:

Becoming Elizabeth Nneka Anionwu

Letter from my mother, 14 March 1972:

> *I can understand you wanting to know about him, if only because your friends are bound to ask questions about your nationality, etc. And if you are mixing with Nigerian people, you just might, by some wild coincidence, meet him, or people who know him. But although I have given you all the information I can, such as it is, I would advise you against making any effort to trace him. At this stage it could have the effect of causing embarrassment to him and his family, and I can't see that any good would come of it.*

This advice from my mother was well-intentioned but it would be ignored, as the letter contained the crucial information that I had needed to know for so long – the name of my father.

> *I have meant for some time to tell you about your father, but as you say, it isn't easy here. He is a Nigerian from Lagos.* [His hometown was in fact Onitsha in south-eastern Nigeria.] *His full name is Lawrence Odiatu Victor Anionwu. He used to be known as Lawrence, or Laurie, among his English friends, but preferred to use his Nigerian name, Odiatu Anionwu.*

It was such a strange sensation, seeing the surname of my father for the very first time, and uppermost in my mind was how I should pronounce it. My mother continued:

I met him when I was at college. I was nineteen at the time. He was quite a bit older. He had been studying law in England for some years and was on the point of being called to the Bar. Shortly after obtaining his final qualifications to practise as a barrister, he returned to Nigeria, permanently. He had a great love of his own country and had no wish to stay in England.

I didn't tell him about you until it was too late for him to alter his arrangements about going home. By that time, I had realised that his feelings about me were less serious than I had imagined and I was just an episode in his life. We did exchange a few letters after his return to Nigeria. Some years later he married a Nigerian girl. I was married to your stepfather by that time. The last I heard from him must be about twenty years ago. He was living in Lagos then and, from what I know of his plans, it seems reasonable to suppose that he is still there.

This letter must have been difficult to write, as it would have brought back such a painful period of my mother's life. Much later, when I obtained her correspondence with Father Hudson's Care, I realised that this account differed with how she had written about it at the time – in this letter to me there is no mention of my parents' engagement or of her plans to join my father in Nigeria.

Apart from noting my father's full name at the back of my diary, I did nothing else with the information for three months. This was probably down to its psychological impact, but also because I was unsure how to proceed. It was unsettling and tumultuous at the same time, and it didn't occur to me to even discuss it with close friends. But I was determined to make enquiries about him, with the huge hope that we might even meet one day.

I pondered over who might be the best person to help me unearth the Nigerian origin of the Anionwu name. Due to the Biafran War, I became aware of three main ethnic groups in Nigeria, but later discovered that there were well over 250 others. Could his surname be Igbo, Hausa-Fulani or Yoruba, or was it from one of the many other groups? There was no internet in the 1970s to help me. More importantly, I had no contact with Nigerians at this time and my Black friends were mainly of Caribbean origin.

Much of my local social life was spent at the Caribbean Overseas Association club, or COA, that used to be based in Acton High Street. It became a meeting place for people like me who were involved with the Saturday School. It was also the HQ for a steel drum band and their rehearsals. One person who regularly attended was John Roberts, a barrister from Sierra Leone, who in 1975 became the first Black person to be made Head of Chambers and the first to be appointed a Queen's Counsel in 1988. Married to a nurse, he also taught Nigerian law students.

I decided to show him my father's name in the hope that he might recognise which part of Nigeria it originated from. It had taken me until the evening of Monday, 10 June 1972, three weeks before my twenty-fifth birthday, to work up to asking John the question. John answered that he wasn't sure, but he promised to investigate further and get back to me. I assumed that this would entail a discussion with some of his law students.

On Wednesday, just two days later, he phoned me at the clinic in Wembley, where I was catching up with some health visiting paperwork. He told me that he had found my father and had already spoken to him. I was in a total state of shock. All I could say was: 'What, you've spoken to my father in Nigeria?' His reply was even more extraordinary: 'No, in London, in Palmers Green.'

I felt dizzy and faint; it was all so sudden and unbelievable. John gave me my father's phone number and said that he was expecting me to call him. That is about all I can remember of the conversation and I'm not even sure whether I thanked him. Much later on, it occurred to me that I hadn't even asked John how on earth he had managed to locate my father so quickly. My assumption that it was through one of his Nigerian law students proved incorrect. At the time, John would occasionally collect his ten-year-old son from school. The Nigerian mother of one of his friends would also be waiting, so John decided to show her my father's name. To his amazement she said that her husband was an Enwonwu and related to my father's wife. They were currently living in London and she gave John his details.

While stunned at this development, I didn't waste any time; I immediately phoned the number he had given me. When I asked to speak to Mr Anionwu, the man at the other end said, 'Speaking,' and I heard my father's voice for the first time. I can't remember the gist of the conversation, except that it resulted in an invitation to visit him and his wife the next day.

So as my diary notes, I 'met F' on the evening of Thursday, 15 June 1972. He and his wife, Regina, lived in a three-bedroomed semi-detached house in Palmers Green in the north London borough of Enfield. It was just off the North Circular Road and it was an effort to keep focused while travelling by scooter in the rush hour along this extremely busy dual carriageway. Pulling up outside the house, the nerves kicked in, and I could feel the butterflies in my stomach. I was both anxious and excited as, after taking a very deep breath, I knocked on the front door. A short, rotund, bespectacled and very dark-skinned man opened it, and I knew immediately it was my father. He beamed at me, looked me up and down, hugged me, stood back, gazed at me again, smiled and said, 'Welcome!' I can still remember the sensation of his warm embrace and the tears that came to my eyes.

It was as though those tears completely washed away my mother's concerns (and mine, to a lesser extent) that tracing him would result in rejection and embarrassment. My father's wife, Regina, also came to the door and said hello, then stared at me for what seemed like a very long time. We all entered the house and Regi, as my father called her, went to prepare a meal while he took me into the sitting room. There, he took out some photographs and showed me pictures of when he was a student at Cambridge and an ambassador in Rome. Looking at one of him wearing white cricket gear, he told me how much he loved all types of sport. He asked me about my mother, and I told him she was fine. Then he wanted to know all about my career to date and seemed to be very proud of my achievements.

Regi called us into the dining room and we sat down for my first introduction to Nigerian food. It was okra (ladies' fingers) stew with pounded yam, which looked like mashed potato. I was invited to eat it using a knife and fork, although I noticed that my father dipped his hand in water before scooping a portion of yam and stew into his mouth. The first spoonful of the okra stew made me gag because it was so slimy and there was laughter around the table. Something else was offered, but I refused as I wanted to try this new dish – and I am very pleased that I persevered, as it is now one of my favourites. But the one that comes top is egusi soup, made from ground melon seeds, crayfish and much more. (Other Nigerian dishes I've thoroughly come to enjoy include jollof rice, fried plantains, or dodo, and moin moin – a spicy, steamed bean pudding.)

How to address my father was my first problem, so I called him Lawrence, as I wasn't ready or brave enough to start calling him Dad – it just felt too strange, as I had simply never had a father figure. The first few letters he wrote to me were also signed Lawrence. But after a few visits, my stepmother Regi took me aside, saying that I shouldn't be calling him Lawrence as he was my father, so from then on I started to call him Dad. I later discovered that my father and his wife had lost their only child in infancy, a daughter called Genevieve. It was clearly a major cause of distress and stigma for a woman to be childless, which must have been exacerbated for Regi on discovering that her husband had other children. I was his eldest child and there were another five children by three different Nigerian women, some of whom I would meet.

Meeting my father that first time was an incredible experience, but obviously full of emotions. Both he and his wife tried to make me feel at home, inviting me to come and visit again whenever I wished, but it wasn't until three weeks later on Saturday, 8 July, six days after my birthday, that I saw them again – and only after my stepmother had called wondering why I hadn't been in touch since my first visit. It was all probably too much for me and, in all honesty, the easiest strategy was to hibernate.

On the second visit, my father recognised my keen interest in politics. He seemed delighted at my wish to learn more about the history of Nigeria, particularly the Biafra War – so much so that for my birthday present, he bought me a copy of journalist John de St Jorre's newly published book, *The Nigerian Civil War*, inscribing it: 'Happy birthday and in remembrance of June 15th, Lawrence 1972.' A more recent publication that has also helped me to understand the background of this horrendous conflict is Chinua Achebe's *There Was a Country: A Personal History of Biafra* (2012).

It was at this second visit that I met my uncle Sunday, my father's youngest brother. He was with his wife, Joy, and four young children, and he invited me later that day to come back with his family to their flat near Finsbury Park. It soon became a home from home for me as it was so welcoming and hospitable, and I loved the youngsters: Charlie, Jenny, Tony and baby John. Time spent there became a very important way of introducing me to Igbo food, culture and Nigerian family life. They invited me to birthday parties in their home and to community events such as weddings. This was a gradual introduction to both my wider family and the large Onitsha community in London.

It was at this time that my father told me that I had a sixteen-year-old half-brother called Emmanuel (or Emma), who was in a private school in Hampshire. He was clearly concerned about his son's poor progress in subjects such as English and the fact he needed to resit examinations. As my father was due to return to Nigeria, he asked me to visit the school, talk to his teachers and let him know what they had to say. So off to Hampshire I went, and met Emma for the first time and spoke to his teachers.

The visit must have been somewhat disconcerting for

him, particularly when I fed back the negative comments from his main tutor. He shrugged off my offer to help him when in London for his holidays and wasn't too happy when I persevered and organised some additional tuition. We never became close friends, but I kept in touch with him – more out of a sense of duty to my father than anything else. Emma was incredibly arrogant, but at least he was happy with the records I gave him as presents after discovering his craze for songs by Barry White.

My father was impressed with how I responded to his request for help with Emma, and it seemed to further cement our relationship. Initially, I was shy around my father and rarely offered my own opinions. But one day he made a remark about current affairs (remember, he was a diplomat and seemingly part of the Establishment, and I was a left-wing radical) that I totally disagreed with and, before knowing it, I had responded quite vigorously with my own views. He was absolutely delighted, saying it was clear that I had been biting my tongue for some time and that it was enjoyable and enlightening for us to debate.

We then started to talk more freely about a variety of matters, and he used to ask me questions about the current British political scene and other subjects. However, I never felt confident enough to ask about his relationship with my mother. Basic things, such as how did they meet? What did they see in each other? How long did they know each other for? What did they do together?

Any child is curious about the history of their parents, and I have sometimes thought about why they didn't stay together and the forces that stopped them. They had been engaged and planned to go to Nigeria, but what sort of life did they envisage out there, given the obstacles they faced? It makes me think of the 2016 film *A United Kingdom*, which was set in the year after they met. The story of Seretse Khama, heir to the throne of Bechuanaland (later Botswana, of which he was president), who studied law in London, and his white British wife, Ruth Williams Khama, it shows how difficult even making a phone call was back then, and the huge political and emotional ramifications of an African leader marrying a white woman.

The fact was that my parents did communicate with each other and the letters from Nazareth House show that my mum gradually realised the relationship wasn't as strong as she thought it was. When he went back to Nigeria, they had been engaged and my mother was planning to go over and live with him once he'd got things settled, but then life took over and they both married other people. My father did tell me that in 1960, he came over for a course and was studying in London. He had tried to contact my mother, but sadly her family had moved house by then and he could no longer contact her or me.

Chapter 28:

My Father

My father was born in Onitsha, an extremely large market town on the eastern banks of the River Niger in the south-eastern state of Anambra. Across the river is the town of Asaba, and the magnificent Niger Bridge connects the two. Historically, Onitsha comprised the traditional community of Inland Town and Onitsha Waterside. Inland Town (Enu-Onicha) is composed of many villages or quarters, and the Anionwu family hails from one called Ogboli Eke. They come under the heading of Nwanna Ugwulu and the sub-heading of Okagbue Oduah. Anionwu then sits within a group of names that includes Amechi Agha, Agbapuonwu Ojiba, Uyanwa Ijagwo, Ifenu Omodi, Onwualu Agba, Ofokansi Nwalie, Chugbo Akwue, Egbuniwe and Nnosa.[1]

My father's entry in the 1943 admissions register to Trinity Hall, Cambridge says: 'Born on the 5th May 1918, the son of Julius Olisa Anionwu of New Market Road, Onitsha, Nigeria.' However, the date of birth on both his death certificate and burial programme is recorded as 5 May 1921, making him three years younger. This tallies with the record of his admission to Lincoln's Inn in November 1946, which gives his age as twenty-five. (I am extremely grateful to all of my Anionwu relatives for providing me with so much information about the family, in particular my cousins Joy and Osita.)

194

My grandfather, Akunne Julius Olisa Osakwe Anionwu, worked at the United African Company (UAC) Ltd in Onitsha. I was informed that he was 'on the quiet side, with impeccable character but quick-tempered' and had fifteen children by four wives. His first wife, my grandmother, was Madam Hanna Echiana Anionwu, née Ejor, from Umuaroli village. The eldest of her four children was my Auntie C, Cecilia Nneka Nnabuenyi Ikeme (1915–1997), followed by my father and then uncles Akunne Frederick Chike (1924–1994) and Onoenyi Sylvester Sunday Onyekwelu (1925–2005).

According to cousin Joy, the daughter of Auntie C: 'Your father did not believe in anybody but my mum because their mother died when they were very young. My mother, being a girl, married very early and was like a guardian to all of them because, by then, their parents were dead and everybody lived with her. This included your dad until he went to read Law at Cambridge and Uncle Sunday before he also left for England.'

My grandfather's brother was Simon Anionwu, who had four wives and a total of twelve children. I came to know two of his sons very well from when they were in London; uncles Akudo from his second wife and Obiozor from his third. I was fortunate enough to meet many of these generations of Anionwu relatives, most of whom are now deceased.

Several family members had been authorised to purchase a traditional Onitsha Ozo title. The Ozo title elevates a man to a high social position and bestows on him the right to officiate as traditional priest on family shrines. The Ozo title society for men is called Agbale Nze. Uncle Chike was known as 'Akunne' and Uncle Sunday as 'Ononenyi'. Otu Odu was the equivalent titled society for women and also required a considerable outlay of money. Auntie Cecilia was addressed as 'Nnabueyi' and her daughter, cousin Joy, is 'Ugobueze', while several female relatives chose the title 'Amalunweze'. My father had never been interested in buying one, even though he was often encouraged (and also teased) by Ozo-titled men that he was wealthy enough to do so. The Ozo title was the level below the Ndichie Chiefs (red cap chiefs), who are a council of ministers appointed by and to advise the Obi, or king, of Onitsha.

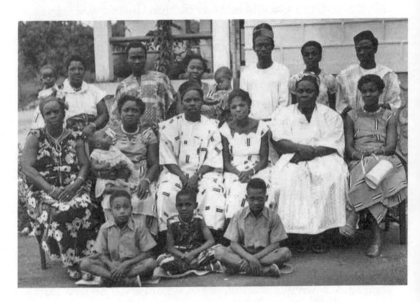

Dad, Regi and the Anionwu family, Onitsha, 1950s.

From all accounts, my father was a very bright child and loved playing football and hockey. He started his education at the Holy Trinity Primary School, Onitsha, before travelling to Lagos for his secondary education at King's College. (He returned to Onitsha for a short spell as a tutor at Christ the King College.) Then, in 1942, in the midst of the Second World War, he sailed to the UK via the Caribbean, travelling with other students including his very good friend Mr Albert Osakwe.

Dad commenced his law studies at Trinity Hall, Cambridge, in 1943. Records show that he achieved a third in both parts of his exams. (While Dad studied at Cambridge, the 2013 book *Black Oxford* by Pamela Roberts explores the long-standing connection between scholars from Africa, the US and the Caribbean, and Oxford. In the nineteenth century, missionary schools educated students for university while, later on, countries including Guyana, Sierra Leone and Ghana all established elite schools that recognised the same curricula as Britain's public schools. Scholarships were also established encouraging Commonwealth students to travel to Britain to study at university.)

In 1946, he proceeded to Lincoln's Inn to complete a Master of Arts degree followed by an LLB degree. They list him as 'having been admitted on 18 November 1946 aged twenty-five, having previously been at Trinity Hall, Cambridge'. I find this date extremely interesting, as I was born eight months later.

His address is given as New Market Road, Onitsha, Nigeria, and his father is listed as Julius Osakwe Anionwu, retired merchant. Lawrence was called to the Bar on 26 January 1949. Trinity Hall also holds correspondence about him studying for twelve months at the Imperial Defence College, now the Royal College of Defence Studies, in Belgrave Square, London – which he was expected to complete on 16 December 1960. A few months earlier, on 1 October, Nigeria had obtained its independence from Britain. I would have been thirteen years of age at the time and living with my grandmother in Wallasey.

Dad returned to Nigeria in 1949, two years after my birth, where he set up thriving law practices in the northern city of Jos and in Onitsha. In 1957, he was appointed a Senior Crown Counsel in the Eastern Nigeria Civil Service, and, in 1958, the Federal Government appointed him Nigerianisation Officer in preparation for independence in 1960. On his return from studies in London, he was appointed the first Nigerian Permanent Secretary to the Minister of External Affairs.

In 1963, he travelled to Rome to take up the post of Nigeria's first Ambassador to Italy. Here, he lived with Regi and his children Emmanuel and Florence, both born to local women he had met when working as a lawyer in Jos. Years before, Auntie C became aware of their existence, travelled to the north of Nigeria and obtained permission from their mothers for the children to live with her at Onitsha. (It wasn't until 2021 that I was to make contact with my sister, as she married an Italian and remained in the country.)

In 1966, my father was transferred to London to take up the post of High Commissioner. This didn't happen for reasons that I have never understood, but which must have been related to the terrible events unfolding in Nigeria. This same year had witnessed deadly interethnic military coups and the slaughter of thousands of Igbo civilians in the north.

On 30 May 1967, Colonel Emeka Ojukwu, the military governor of the Eastern Region of Nigeria, declared independence of the south-eastern region, naming it the Republic of Biafra. Less than two months later saw the outbreak of the tragic Biafra or Civil War that lasted from 6 July 1967 to 15 January 1970. I never asked him the question: 'What did you do in the war, Daddy?' But while writing this book, I trawled the internet to see whether there was any information and came across two interesting items.

The first was that the UK National Archives held information entitled: 'Activities of Mr. L O U (*sic*) Anionwu, 01/01/1967–31/12/1967', which both excited and intrigued me greatly. Imagine my surprise to discover that the document was a copy of three typed A3 pages of a confidential 700-word note of a meeting my father had had on 14 June 1967 at the Foreign and Commonwealth Office (FCO). This was just a mere three weeks before the outbreak of the conflict. It is also weird to realise that I wouldn't have been too far away, completing my second year of nursing studies in Paddington.

My father spoke with Sir Saville Garner, Permanent Undersecretary and Head of the Diplomatic Service. The confidential record of the meeting was written for his superior, Sir Morrice James, then Deputy Undersecretary of State at the Commonwealth Office. It was also copied to the Minister of State (then George Thomas), Mr Norris (Sir Eric Norris, Assistant Undersecretary for West, East & South Africa) and Sir David Hunt, who had recently been appointed High Commissioner in Lagos. The latter, according to foreign policy author Mark Curtis, had written in a memo to London just two days before: '[The] only way . . . of preserving unity [*sic*] of Nigeria is to remove Ojukwu by force.' He believed that Ojukwu was committed to remaining the ruler of an independent state and that British interests lay in firmly supporting the Federal Military Government. Curtis argues that previously confidential papers reveal that Britain's true interest lay in protecting their oil interests.

Gardner's note of the meeting with my father starts by recalling that he had last entertained him: '. . . when he was (as we thought at the time) about to become High Commissioner in London just over a year ago. He told me that when the London appointment fell through owing to Ogundipe coming here, he was offered the Embassy in Moscow and subsequently the Embassy in Brazil, but he had declined both of these.'

Many years later, I acquired a copy of *West Africa* magazine dated 25 February 1967, where there was an announcement that my father had been named Ambassador to Brazil. Garner continues: 'I gathered that in fact he had remained technically on leave but in receipt of full pay and had returned to the Eastern Region. He explained that he was anxious to keep aloof from both sides in the dispute, since if he made contact with either he would be suspect to the other.'

Brigadier-General Babafemi Ogundipe had been chief of staff and de facto vice-president of Nigeria following the military coup on 16 January 1966 by Major-General Johnson Aguiyi-Ironsi. Prior to this, Ogundipe had been the Nigerian military attaché in London. The period of Aguiyi-Ironsi's rule was extremely short due to his overthrow and assassination on 29 July 1966.

My father said that the purpose of his visit to London was to make alternative holiday arrangements for his two children at school in the UK. The plan had been for them to return to Nigeria for the summer holiday, but this was no longer possible in the current situation. Garner asked him about the conditions in Nigeria and he replied that any break-up of Nigeria would be a tragedy, the view of most educated Nigerians, including those in the Eastern Region. He thought that the ideal would be a 'loose federation'. My father commented that the 'tragedy was the appalling massacre in the North last year and the dispossessing of so many Igbo families had caused a bitterness throughout the Eastern Region, which it is impossible to ignore. There was no family which did not have some member who had been either killed or dispossessed.'

My father didn't believe that Ojuwku was unreasonable or unduly ambitious: '. . . he was, on the contrary, a well-educated and moderate person who had everything to lose from the materialist point of view in a row with the Federal Government since he had a fortune of over half a million pounds in investments outside the Eastern Region.' He argued that sanctions would never succeed in bringing Ojuwku to heel and that military force would be disastrous. My father was then asked how he thought a solution could be found. He replied that he saw no prospect of Gowon and Ojuwku coming together and he couldn't identify anyone in Nigeria 'big enough to be able to influence a settlement on the right lines'. As a result, he thought that some outside influence would have to be brought to bear. Garner pointed out the difficulty of imposing a solution from outside, unless the person was acceptable to both sides.

My father recognised that 'it would not be desirable for the British to take any initiative and, indeed, thought it would be better for white faces not to be too prominent'. He felt that there might be a role for the Commonwealth secretariat but wondered whether they had sufficient prestige. He suggested that they should associate with 'somebody with a reputation like Kenyatta to carry the necessary weight'. The note of the meeting ended: 'Mr Anionwu concluded with, I thought, a rather forced optimism that, if only the present difficulties could be got over, there was a splendid future for Nigeria and no reason why the various Regions should not work together in what could still remain a Nigerian nation.'

The second item I found online concerned a US National Broadcasting Company (NBC) clip about a 'Biafra War Press

Conference', which was never broadcast. It was filmed at London's Mayfair Hotel on 20 June 1967, six days after my father's meeting at the Foreign and Commonwealth Office. It describes the clip as a:

PRESS CONFERENCE WITH M T MBU; A MEMBER OF THE SECESSIONIST STATES EXECUTIVE COUNCIL & CHAIRMAN OF THE PUBLIC SERVICES COMMISSION; & LAWRENCE ANIONWU; FORMER PERMANENT SECRE-TARY OF THE NIGERIAN EXTERNAL AFFAIRS MINISTRY IN LAGOS. MBU COMMENTS ON THE PROBABILITY OF ENGLAND RECOGNIZING THE NEW STATE OF BIAFRA. ANIONWU COMMENTS ON THE PROBLEM OF ISSUING PASSPORTS TO DIPLOMATS. ORDINARY CITIZENS CAN CONTINUE TO USE NIGERIAN PASSPORTS; HE SAYS.

The now deceased Chief Matthew Tawo Mbu was an eminent politician who had also been the first high commissioner for Nigeria in the UK between 1955 and 1959. During the war, he was appointed the Biafran foreign minister from 1967 to 1970.

Anionwu relatives later informed me that Dad had been in Biafra for the duration of the war. He had worked for the Republic of Biafra as a Permanent Secretary, first in the Ministry of Labour and then in the Ministry of Works. At one point he had been living and working in Aba when the town was the target of a major bombing raid on 21 December 1967. Fortunately, he was at his office, as the kitchen of his home received a direct hit. Regi was in the lounge with a guest, but neither was injured. Less fortunate that day were the many people killed in the market and at Onyejiaka Hospital, including the owner, Dr Augustine Onyejiaka. After the war ended, Dad retired from public office and settled in London with Regi. So in June 1972, and two and a half years after the war ended, my father and I were to meet for the very first time. One of the photographs he gave me that day showed him greeting Pope Paul VI following his appointment as Nigeria's first ever Ambassador to Italy.

My mother was genuinely delighted to hear that all was going well, even though she was clearly shocked that I had found my father so quickly. I wrote to my great-aunt Kate to tell her that I had met up with my father. She received my letter on 5 September 1972, which happened to be her eighty-third birthday! Her reaction to my news was very moving:

> It was an unexpected treat, like an extra birthday treat . . . Meeting with your father and discovering that you liked him and were acceptable to him was quite an experience. I am happy for you. It is good to feel that you really belong, and I am sure you will enjoy a stay in Nigeria when the time comes. Although we do not have any physical contact, I never forget you. You always have a place in my prayers.

Chapter 29:

Nigeria

Dad returned to live in Nigeria in 1972 and wrote to let me know that he had arrived at Onitsha on 24 November. The destructive legacy of the war was still being felt. The main post office had been completely damaged and the smaller local one wasn't coping, so there were delays in receiving my letters, which didn't always arrive in the order they were sent.

He went back to his legal practice and became active in village affairs. Relatives told me that in choosing not to take the Ozo title, my father may have been following in the footsteps of one of his role models, Sir Louis Nwachukwu Mbanefo. He was a renowned lawyer, jurist and Chief Justice of the Eastern Region of Nigeria. Equally prominent was my father's friend Chief Atanda Fatayi Williams, a colleague at Trinity College and former Chief Justice of Nigeria.

It hadn't taken me long to decide that I did indeed want to visit Nigeria as soon as possible. I was determined to travel to Nigeria, but despite not having much money, it never occurred to me to ask my father for help in purchasing the air ticket. The funds came in a rather unusual way following a scooter crash at a roundabout as I was nearing my workplace one Friday morning in September 1972. My father had been extremely worried about me and insisted that I recuperate at his home in Palmers Green. The subsequent award of £150 compensation paid for my Egyptair flight to Nigeria in July of the following year.

By then I had once again moved, this time to West Ealing. Here, I shared a spacious flat with three other women for four years. My own bed-sitting room was large enough to have both a bed and a sofa, so Dad stayed with me when he came to London. He slept in my bed while I used the sofa and, although it was comfortable, sleep didn't come easily as he snored loudly, just like me.

During one of his trips the phone rang; it was my mother with a query about a medical clue in a crossword puzzle, and I realised I had the chance to close this circle of connection. I quietly asked her if she would like to speak to him and, while surprised, she agreed. My dad was also happy to talk to her, so I left them alone to chat together, as I didn't want to overhear the conversation – there was no curiosity in me and I felt that it had to be a very private conversation between the pair of them. I never asked either of them about their one and only discussion, but was pleased that I had linked them together again and neither of them were upset with me. I was really happy I'd made it happen.

In July 1973, a year after our first meeting, my father wrote: 'I am glad you have been to see your mum and that she is happy about your proposed visit to Nigeria.' Then he thanked me for books that I had sent him via Regi, especially *The Man Died: Prison Notes of Wole Soyinka*, adding that he was better informed for having read it. Published in 1971, it recounted Soyinka's 27-month imprisonment without trial during the Biafra War and the searing mental trauma of solitary confinement.

At the end of July, I set off on my first trip to Nigeria. Stepping off the plane in Lagos on 31 July, the sweltering heat wrapped itself around my body as though enveloping me with the warmth of my Nigerian family. The country was under military rule and led by General Yakubu Gowon, the same regime that had taken over after the July 1966 coup and assassination of Major-General Aguiyi-Ironsi. Gowon's image was visible on posters throughout the airport and armed soldiers were everywhere.

The trip was mind-blowing, enjoyable from start to finish, with a few unsettling but pleasant surprises in between. My father had written to let me know that he would meet the flight at Lagos, which was then the capital of Nigeria. The plan was that we would stay a few days with a very good friend of his, Mr George Nicol, a solicitor and businessman who lived in the smart Lagos neighbourhood of South West Ikoyi. We would then travel nearly 300 miles by car to Onitsha, via Benin City.

It was with great excitement that I looked around for my father in the airport's arrival lounge. I eagerly absorbed the sounds, colours and smells that assailed me. He was nowhere to be seen, and I waited and waited patiently while new arrivals came and went. I knew nobody and had no telephone number except my father's at Onitsha. An unexpected boost to my morale was that several members of staff immediately recognised the name of my father and took pity on me. Showing one of them his phone number, I asked where the nearest phone box was so that I could call and see if the family could tell me where he was. They very gently laughed, saying it was difficult enough to get through to Lagos telephone numbers, never mind as far away as Onitsha.

When it became late, they suggested that I should stay in a nearby hotel; if my father turned up, they would let him know where I was. They found a cab for me and warned the driver to take good care of me. Once in bed, I just cried my eyes out for ages, because this was not how I envisioned my first evening in Nigeria. Exhausted, I fell fast asleep before being woken by the telephone ringing in my room. To my utter joy, I heard my father's voice saying that he was in the lobby downstairs. He asked me to pack my case and meet him in the foyer – I was dressed in a flash. It transpired that he had misunderstood the time of my arrival (a mix-up between 24-hour and twelve-hour timing). Anyway, all was sorted and I was extremely relieved as we drove off to his friend's house.

We stayed there for a few days and I was made truly welcome, but the experience proved to be a major culture shock. Mr Nicol was a rotund and jovial man, obviously quite well off and had a servant called Friday. I was starting to realise that people can be called by the days of the week, as I had an Uncle Sunday, so another day didn't surprise me. What did, though, was the way in which Mr Nicol would bark his orders out for Friday, who was a middle-aged man. In response, he would come running in shouting, '*Sah!*' and sometimes his boss would just want him to turn the television on or get him a drink. This seemed crazy and was quite upsetting but, when I discussed it with my father, he said this is a different way of life, although not everyone acted like that.

Everyone was extremely friendly and very keen to show me parts of Lagos life that I wanted to see, such as the market. Cloth was bought for me, which was used at Onitsha to make my first traditional wrapper and blouse, which made me feel great and was part of how my family wanted me to connect with my Igbo identity. It was a present that made me feel more of a member of my family and community. I was accepted and welcomed, no questions asked – my Irish-heritage family had done their best for me, but they'd been overcome with fear and stigma. In Nigeria, I was struck by the openness and attitude of 'What are you worried about?'

When I read Barack Obama's 1995 memoir, *Dreams from My Father*, it resonated with me because when he went to Kenya to visit his father's birthplace he, too, felt utterly accepted. I was twenty-six when I first visited the continent of Africa and he was twenty-seven. We both returned with a possibly over-romantic view of our trips, but both had the sensation of coming home. Obama's grandmother spoke Luo and no English, and she was pained that he was unable to speak to her. He asked his half-sister to explain that 'It's hard to find time in the States. Tell her how busy I am.' Her translated reply was that she understood, but that 'a man can never be too busy to know his own people'. This completely reflected my own experiences of being unable to speak Igbo.

It was wonderful to have time with my father during that long drive from Lagos, and en route he pointed out landmarks and the different types of tropical vegetation. He laughed at some of the rather naive comments I made on the journey. As an example, I couldn't see anything similar to the yellow AA boxes in Britain that you would call from should you have a breakdown. He said, 'No, there's no such thing. You just make sure your car is serviced very well before you set out on your journey.' He added that if you did break down there are mechanics galore, and one would emerge from the bush onto the main road.

The scenery was incredible and so lush that I just sat back and thoroughly enjoyed the drive. Hawkers on the road would wave baskets of fruit and other food, and my father would occasionally pull over and quickly haggle the price down. We stopped off at Benin in the Mid-Western Region, and I still can recall those dusty red roads. We stayed with my cousin Vicky and her family, and she took some time off work at the university to take us to the local sights, including the palace of the Oba of Benin.

We then continued our journey along the very straight road to Asaba. My father merely told me that we were going to visit a friend's house in Asaba; he could be a man of few words. While he had a great sense of humour, I realised that he would only tell you things when he was ready. As we drove into the compound, I saw people dancing with what looked like sticks with black feathers on them. They were waving them around, and as we got nearer the house the sound of drumming became louder and I could see people holding a photograph of a man. I turned to my father in the car and asked, 'What's happening, is it a wedding?' to which he replied, 'No, it's a funeral.' My shocked face said it all.

When we got out of the car, my father was greeted by a huge number of people. He introduced me as his daughter, and it was quite amusing to watch the reaction. It was clear that although a few were already aware, most weren't – but while surprised, their unanimous reaction was huge smiles followed by a warm embrace. At some point he introduced me to a cousin and asked her to look after me. She took me into a room where women in black dresses were sitting around a four-poster bed. Lo and behold, there was a dead man dressed in a suit and lying in state on the bed. There was a big fan hanging from the ceiling, whirring away, and people were also waving traditional fans to keep cool. As a nurse, I was obviously used to seeing dead bodies, but I had never seen one laid out in a house. Later on, we went out into the compound, where suddenly I saw a group of people running while carrying the coffin, and every so often throwing it up into the air. My cousin explained that it was a ritual that symbolised the soul of the deceased person's struggle in leaving the body.

A huge crowd payed homage to this well-known personality as the coffin was lowered into the grave. One contrast with a British funeral was the level of noise: there was a lot of weeping, wailing and shouting and, to my horror, one particular woman seemed to be about to leap into the grave. My father, seeing my amazement, tapped my arm and whispered into my ear: 'Don't worry, many of those who scream the loudest loved the person the least.' It certainly relaxed me and, in fact, I had to bite my tongue to avoid laughing. It was comments like this that made me realise we had a very similar sense of humour.

After the funeral, we crossed over the splendid Niger Bridge into Onitsha that had been built in 1965 to replace the ferry crossing. Akunne Abadom, an Onitsha elder in London, recounted many years later how, as a young boy in 1949, he and others went down to the ferry to welcome my father home from his studies in the UK. Unfortunately, they waited in vain as he had returned via Enugu. On all future visits I would continue to be impressed by the stunning view of the Niger Bridge, as it signalled the approach to Onitsha.

The family had decided that it would be best if I stayed with my Auntie C in New Market Road, Onitsha. I later discovered that this was because there were severe tensions between my father and his wife, Regi, and also between Regi and my father's relatives. We went to the house, where I was given the most incredible welcome. I'll never forget it.

My auntie hugged me and generally fussed over me, before showing me off to a host of visitors. I was introduced to her eldest daughter, Nkiru, who took charge of all of my needs when her mother was out of the house. Everybody called me Lizzy (even though I never used this name) and as an elder daughter from Ogboli Eke, I was also addressed as 'Abii' as well as 'Ada'.

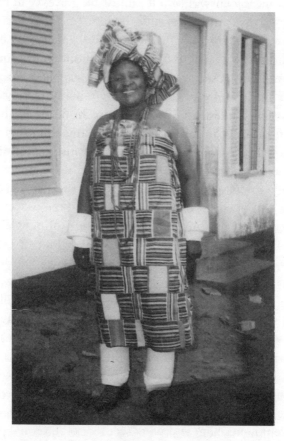

Auntie C.

Auntie C immediately decided that I had to have an Igbo middle name. At that point I had my Catholic names of Elizabeth Mary and my surname was still Furlong. My auntie sat me down with other relatives and had a family discussion, something that was to happen very frequently during my stay. I didn't understand a thing, as it was all in Igbo, but occasionally some of it would be translated. There was no sense of feeling left out, and it proved a useful way of picking up a few Igbo words here and there.

It was decided that my new middle name would be Nneka, the Igbo name of Auntie C. I was extremely touched, as it means 'my mother is supreme' – it seemed a wonderful thing to me. My Nigerian family were always asking about my mother and seemed to recognise how much she had done to bring me up. After no one talking about my father as I grew up, it was so great to find that his family were so interested in my mother and what she'd done for me. The fact they articulated it by saying, 'How is she?' or 'Give your mother our greetings' meant she was part of the conversation.

It was also hilarious to see the reaction of people when I was introduced as 'nwa LOV' – 'the daughter of LOV' (a familiar way of referring to my father). Some people actually realised before they were told. I couldn't believe how many people described me as 'Little Lawrence' or 'Little LOV'. There were also constant observations concerning how much we resembled each other.

I slept like a log that first night at Onitsha, tucked up in a bed covered with a mosquito net. In the morning, three distinct noises woke me – cocks crowing, the sound of highlife music from a nearby shop (both of which I would always enjoy hearing) and what seemed to be several people whispering, either just outside or actually in my bedroom. I peered through the netting with one eye only to see a group of women sitting around my bed quietly talking to each other. What on earth was going on? I was quite shocked that my private space had been invaded.

One of the women saw that I was awake and suddenly ripped back the net and told me they were relatives who wanted to greet me. Shouts and exclamations of '*Chukwu dalo!*' ('Thanks be to God') and '*Ewo!*' ('Oh no!') together with the greetings of '*Nno!*' ('Welcome!') and '*Kedu?*' ('How are you?') were heard from all and sundry. This was also accompanied by lots of hugs, kisses and comments on how much I looked like my father. Then my aunt shooed them all out and showed me where I could do my ablutions before breakfast. In the bath was a large bucket that had been filled with warm water and I showered using the large plastic mug nearby. It was very refreshing, and back in England I still use this method if ever the electric shower isn't working.

My favourite of all the numerous memories of this first trip was being forced to learn a few Igbo words by Ike, a cheeky and sweet eight-year-old. His grandmother, Auntie C (whom he called Mamma), was caring for him. He was the son of my cousin Nnamdi, who was affected by sickle cell anaemia and living in England. Auntie C had apparently asked Ike to teach me some Igbo, and he took on this duty with great gusto. He was also responsible for preparing my breakfast, and he wouldn't let me have a bite of it until I spoke a few words to him in Igbo. This worked like a charm and I quickly learned '*Biko*' ('Please') and '*Dalo*' ('Thank you'), along with many other words, to ensure I got some food along with that first cup of tea of the day. (Ike now lives in England, and his lovely son is footballer Carl Ikeme, who was the goalkeeper for Wolverhampton Wanderers FC until his early retirement in 2017 due to leukaemia; he's now thankfully in remission.)

A more painful souvenir was when it was decided I should have my ears pierced. My auntie and others took me to the compound of a nearby house, where I was asked to sit on a stool. Amid lots of joking and encouraging noises, a woman proceeded to clean and then rub each earlobe, pierce them with a sharp instrument and then insert a piece of black thread through the hole. Fortunately, it was all done very quickly and there were no problems apart from the sting that occurred when women came up from behind and pulled the thread back and forth to keep the hole open. It was all worth it when my father presented me with a lovely set of gold earrings – and I no longer felt out of place as the only woman without pierced ears.

It was wonderful to explore Onitsha. First on the agenda was a visit to Uncle Chike, who was living in the family house in Anionwu Street. On my travels, I noticed that there was still evidence of war-damaged property. In the few quiet periods, I was able to read books purchased at one of the many stalls at Onitsha Market or on the road. So it was that I discovered the works of eminent Igbo authors such as Flora Nwapa's *Efuru* (1966) and *Things Fall Apart* (1958), and *A Man of the People* (1966) by Chinua Achebe.

Although I felt accepted and welcomed in Onitsha, it also quickly became apparent to me that I certainly stood out as a non-local. It wasn't just that my skin was a lighter brown colour, as this isn't that uncommon. It was more my general behaviour, accent and inability to speak Igbo. This frequently led to being referred to as '*oyinbo*', which is a Yoruba word that (while open to debate) is often used to indicate white or fair-skinned foreigners. Children in the market would say it to me in a slightly cheeky and humorous way, but it can sometimes be viewed as a derogatory comment.

I was able to attend a lot of events such as Ozo titles, weddings and yet more funerals. There would always be drumming and dancing by different 'age grades' (people born between a certain period), who would all be wearing the same costumes. There was plenty of food and drink such as palm wine. My camera was kept busy, capturing images of beautifully dressed people, many in traditional robes. There were various rituals, such as the breaking of the kola nut by the most senior titled person at the event. It would then be handed out and, although I really tried, it was much too bitter for me to eat. Then there would be libations, with the pouring of schnapps onto the ground accompanied by prayers to the ancestors and numerous deities.

My father continued to introduce me to family and friends at Onitsha and elsewhere. The hospitality was overwhelming, as it was clear that he was well and truly respected and loved by so many people. He also told me how pleased he was that I was comfortable with meeting so many of them. One day we drove nearly seventy miles to Enugu (which means 'the top of the hill'), the former capital of the Eastern Region and initially for the Federal Republic of Biafra. We visited so many people that I started to lose count. At every home we were constantly offered drinks, followed by a choice of food such as plain or jollof rice, pounded yam, eba (cassava) with fish, chicken, meat, okra or egusi stew.

Bloated after the third meal and being driven to the next destination, I told my dad that it would be impossible to eat any more. He explained that it would be necessary just to have a smaller portion, as it would be very disrespectful to refuse. It proved to be a very useful lesson for the future.

At Onitsha, I met a very good friend of my father for the first time. Mr Albert Osakwe was a former Nigerian ambassador and someone I would often visit in London. When I later remarked that they seemed like young lads having a tremendous time, whether at the Onitsha sports club or on their trips abroad attending Rotary Conventions, my dad said, 'Spot on!' Sadly, in 2003, Mr Osakwe's own security guard murdered him at his home in Onitsha.

Throughout my stay, remarks were made about how pleased people were that I was willing to learn as much as possible, taste new foods and even try to speak a few words of Igbo. The time I had spent in London with my dad and Uncle Sunday and his family was proving very useful, as I had at least tasted some of the traditional foods that were provided at various meals. Many a time I was regaled with stories of children, and even some adults, arriving from Britain who insisted on only eating cornflakes and whatever tinned food they had brought with them in their suitcase.

In between all these visits with my father, the younger generation of relatives took great delight in taking me to parties and clubs. This helped me to relax further, as there was no question of being allowed just to sit down and watch others dance. Weddings were another opportunity to eat, dance and be merry. The range of music I was introduced to was fantastic, from modern to highlife, and the more traditional Igbo sounds. Highlife was my absolute favourite, although some tracks could last fifteen minutes or more, so tough luck if you weren't too enamoured with your dancing partner.

Although I was looking forward to returning home, it was with some sadness that I boarded the plane on 29 August 1973. Back in London, I soon discovered Sterns record shop, which for many years was located behind Warren Street station. It had the most incredible collection of West African and other world music. Over the years, I was able to buy lots of records, including many highlife classics. Favourites included 'Joromi' by Sir Victor Uwaifo, 'Salawe' by Chief Rex Lawson and 'Ije Awele' by Chief Osita Steven Osadebe. Whenever they were played at the parties I attended with my cousins in London, memories would come flooding back of my incredible first trip to Nigeria.

For the first time in my life, I now felt completely accepted and was absolutely thrilled with how I was embraced by so many relatives. Many years later, my cousin Joy revealed that on meeting me, her mum, my beloved Auntie C 'was the happiest person ever. Your presence validated a lot of things for her and the whole family. She said that you are the blueprint of your father and that says a lot.' It was really heartening that my presence didn't engender feelings of stigma due to illegitimacy or the colour of my skin. My father's letter to me dated 8 October 1973 sums this up and was an utter joy to read: 'I am delighted that at least you enjoyed your brief stay at home. One result it has undoubtedly accomplished is your introduction to the family and by that I mean those who really mattered. They, too, are really happy. Left to them, you should just start to work here.'

Chapter 30:

Family

The most significant impact of my visit to Nigeria was my desire to go and work there and hence to start to learn Igbo – a wish shared by my family in Onitsha, but not by my father. While he was pleased, he sounded a huge note of caution in pointing out that, not having grown up in Nigeria, I was unaware of the intricacies of life there and would be eaten alive. He explained that contacts were absolutely vital and that mine were few and far between. Therefore, the best plan would be for me to wait until I could work in Nigeria at a very senior level.

At the time, I thought my career was going reasonably well, having completed my nurse training, undertaken seven months' midwifery experience, lived in France for nine months and now being qualified as a health visitor. I didn't have any further ambitions, apart from doing a short course in tropical diseases at the London School of Hygiene & Tropical Medicine. This was completed successfully in early 1974, six months after returning from that first visit to Nigeria. So when my father sat me down one day and asked me how I could progress in my job – what advancement was possible? – I wasn't expecting him to be so interested.

I know today that the NHS and other professions place real emphasis on mentoring and career guidance, but I'd had nothing. Him asking me this question made me focus on the different pathways I could pursue, such as management, clinical or education. The last of the three appeared more appropriate for me. I loved teaching, whether in health promotion sessions with parents in the home and clinic or with pupils at the local secondary school. My father said, 'Well, how can you become a tutor? Maybe you had better look into that.'

My first reaction was that I was far too inexperienced, but lo and behold, my application to do a one-year community nurse tutor course was successful. It was organised in collaboration with the Royal College of Nursing and the University of Surrey and started in the autumn of 1974. My fees were paid courtesy of a Hospital Savings Association (HSA) Scholarship. Both of my parents were extremely proud of how my career was progressing and of the news of my admission to the community nurse tutor course. I remember a congratulatory phone call from Mum. Dad wrote: 'I shall pass on the good news to the rest of the family. You know how happy they will be.'

The next few years were marked by a deepening relationship with both of my parents. I was never to feel any warmth towards Ken, and there were times when I couldn't understand why my mother stayed with him. I still had the vivid memory of her trying to get away from him by going to the police station with Frank as a baby in a pram, and knowing she wasn't happy. Why did she allow it to go on? A lasting influence it had on me was that I would never allow a man to boss me around. Even a glimmer of authoritarianism or macho behaviour and they were gone. Due to my experience of physical violence, there was no way I was going to let myself be in that situation. Even a slight threat of violence and I would feel a lion roar deep within me.

Fortunately, as I got older I gradually came to realise what she must have gone through in trying to make a home for me. The change in my feelings was helped by the fact that, after I qualified as a nurse and health visitor, she started to open up to me. We would discuss some of her difficulties, either in letters or over the phone, and I also started to make more frequent visits to see her in person. I would go on a Sunday, deliberately arriving when Ken was likely to be at the pub, stay about three or four hours and then drive back to London.

I was also in regular correspondence with my father. The contents of the letters reveal sharp differences in my mother and father's social and economic status and also in their everyday preoccupations. In November 1973, my father mentioned returning to Jos to negotiate a new five-year tenancy agreement. At the top of his notepaper, which was headed 'Anionwu & Co, Legal Practitioners & Notaries Public', he addressed me as 'My dear Nneka' and signed off 'Lots of love, Dad'. In preparing to re-establish his practice, he requested that I obtain new legal stationery for him headed 'LOV Anionwu, MA, LLB (Cantab), idc, Barrister-at-Law, Lincoln's Inn'.

In March 1974, he wrote to say how sorry he was to hear what Mum had been through as a result of the economic situation. He also apologised that the promised air ticket for a summer trip to Nigeria wasn't possible due to cash flow problems as a result of overinvesting. Selling some of his land in Lagos, he continued, should ease this. By the following March, he had moved into his new house in Awka Road, just within the boundaries of Ogboli Eke village. As armed robbers were still about, there was now an Alsatian dog for increased security.

In the meantime, Mum had clearly been experiencing severe financial hardship. In February 1974, she apologised about being unable to attend my HSA scholarship award ceremony at Kensington Town Hall, due to lack of funds. It caused me sadness and annoyance, as I would have sent money for the rail fare if I had been aware of her difficulties. In the same letter, she recounted Ken's drink problem. Two years previously, he'd fought with a neighbour and spent a week in the eye infirmary as a result. His unreasonable behaviour continued, and he was making unfounded accusations about her. One day he had got blind drunk and everyone had walked out, staying overnight at the home of a friend's family. Mum wrote that she had planned to apply for a separation order but didn't, because Ken had said he would be different in the future. My anger, concern and frustration knew no bounds, perhaps as this episode also highlighted the widely different social circumstances of my parents.

Both parents updated me with news of the family, be that in Wolverhampton or Onitsha, and were equally keen that I kept in touch. In November 1973, my father described preparations for the second burial of his uncle Simon, head of the Anionwu/Uyanwa family. This Igbo ritual ensures that the deceased person transitions successfully from a state of torment (*'ita okazi'*) to one of peace and serenity. Each parent wrote about their worries and saw me as someone from whom they were comfortable to seek advice. My father apologised in two separate letters for writing so much about his worries concerning Emma, who was now in the upper sixth and doing two A level subjects. He complained: 'I have no idea whether he succeeded in the O level exams. Please find out for me what it is all about.' By October he sounded a little more hopeful, as Emma told him of my visit to his school in Surrey and our outings on Saturday and Sunday. 'Emma sounds more and more enthusiastic, but I would very much like to see this enthusiasm put into action.'

A totally different anxiety for my father erupted with the onset of a major dispute concerning the famous Onitsha Market. On 10 June 1974, he wrote explaining that the market had burned down and how 'the allocation of stalls grievously offended the entire Onitsha people and they are resolved to fight it. I am the Chairman of the Committee appointed for that purpose.' A full history of the whole affair, entitled *Onitsha Market Crisis*, was written and published in January 1976 by Chief Nnamdi Azikiwe, the Owelle of Onitsha, former President of Nigeria and a close friend of my father.

There is an account of my father being held in detention in November 1974:

> Just before the motion to grant an interim injunction to restrain the first Defendant from opening the Onitsha Main Market was argued, the Police invited Mr L.O.V. Anionwu, leading Counsel of the Plaintiffs, to visit Enugu for a tête-à-tête. Of his own volition, he travelled the sixty-seven miles from Onitsha to Enugu in his personal car and, on arrival there, he was detained without trial. Mr Anionwu was formerly Senior State Counsel, sometime Permanent Secretary in the Federal Ministry of External Affairs and Commonwealth Relations, and one-time Ambassador of Nigeria to Rome. He was detained for three days and no reason has been given for this executive act.

My father never wrote about or discussed this incident with me, although I still have a copy of the front page of a national Nigerian newspaper, the *Daily Times*, dated 29 November

1974. The headline of the article reads, EX-ENVOY ANIONWU DETAINED IN ENUGU.

On 6 March 1975, Dad sent me money to purchase books for his research on the history of Onitsha and the market. One that I was able to buy was *The Gospel on the Banks of the Niger* by missionaries Samuel Crowther and John Christopher Taylor, originally published in 1859. In August 1975, Mum was delighted when Marion and Pam came to stay with me for a holiday in London and, in thanking me for arranging the weekend visit, added that she couldn't afford to get their photos printed yet. In September 1975, Dad reported that the family were overjoyed that Uncle Sunday had now returned to Onitsha after eighteen years' absence.

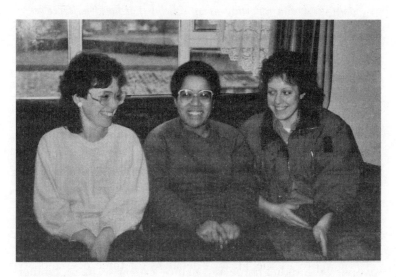

Me with my sisters, Marion and Pam.

In November 1975, Mum started a very long letter to me with: 'I would be glad of your opinion as . . .' She then went on to describe Ken's chronic bronchitis and asthma that would require him to retire due to ill health and explained that 'he wants me to leave work regardless of reducing the family to living on social security. He thinks that it is my duty to put him first and accept this standard of living if necessary, rather than go on working.'

In explaining her resentment, she continued:

What makes me really sick about the prospect of having to resign myself to that sort of existence is the fact that up to now, I have been doing extremely well with the advanced shorthand course that I told you about and I am within reaching distance of getting the job I have always wanted, doing verbatim reporting as an official shorthand writer. I've had to wait over twenty years for the children to grow up before I could go to classes and take the requisite exams, and now this has to happen.

It made me so angry that Ken was putting her in this position – hadn't she done enough for him? I was so pleased she stood up to him and said no, but her distress upset me. Could she never get away from this sense of subservience? It was awful to witness, though I was pleased she was asking for my advice and talking to me about it.

Health problems were gradually starting to affect both of my parents. In October 1974, Mum had had an eight-hour spell of amnesia due to high blood pressure. Given all of her worries, this didn't come as much of a surprise. In September 1975, Dad informed me that he had just been discharged from Iyi-Enu Hospital, five miles outside Onitsha. He had been a patient there for seven days due to pneumonia and high blood pressure, and requested that I obtain some good medicine for the latter and give them to his friend Mr Osakwe.

My social life had by now changed dramatically, as I was frequently socialising with Nigerian relatives and their friends. I had become particularly close to my beautiful cousin Joy, and I have great memories of us meeting up with her friends on Friday evenings in north London. The phone would be busy as they checked out where the weekend parties would be held, usually in flats of students around London. It always surprised me how many people could cram into them, staying well into the early hours of the morning.

Money seemed to flow; it was, after all, the time of the Nigerian oil boom. There was incredible food of jollof rice, and meat, and drink and, in between the dancing, it was possible to catch up with all the gossip. The DJ would always play a mix of records including soul, R&B, reggae and Motown, together with modern Nigerian music – I wasn't allowed to sit down and found it so easy to dance. Often, at about 2 a.m., there would be dancing to the sounds of traditional Igbo music and I would love watching Joy's moves. I started going out with Nigerian boyfriends and photos of the period show me wearing much more fashionable attire. It was really good fun, and Joy really looked after me.

It was at one such party late in 1973 where I met Beje. He was a good-looking guy, very intelligent and proud of his roots. He also had a lovely sense of humour, which is always a huge attraction for me. We had great fun together and visited many friends around the country, as well as going off to Paris for a holiday. He was a member of the Itsekiri ethnic group from the Delta State of Nigeria, and was studying for a master's degree in engineering.

In April 1974, Dad wrote asking about him and thanking me for the photo of the two of us. He also queried whether I had written to Auntie C about him. While on a trip to Nigeria in September 1974, Beje and his brother travelled to Onitsha and had lunch with Regi and Dad. They stayed three hours and he met with Dad's approval: 'I find him very intelligent and interested in current affairs. I like him.' Soon after, Beje came to Wolverhampton to meet Mum and on 3 October 1974, she wrote: 'Hope Beje is well. It was nice meeting him and we all hope he can come again when possible.'

In January 1975, I was pleasantly surprised to receive a letter from his father, a chief from Sapele in Nigeria. 'I have heard about you going out with my son for some time. I am writing to your father today and will go to Onitsha to see him sometime this year. Extend greetings to your mother and I will write to her some time if God permits.' My father wrote to tell me that he did indeed receive the letter and was looking forward to meeting him.

We became engaged, but unfortunately he seemed to feel this gave him a licence to date other women, and I wasn't having any of that. I was up in Scotland on training, and I think Joy alerted me to what he was doing, so by the end of 1975 I'd given him the heave-ho.

Chapter 31:
Professional, Personal, Political

While I still wanted to work in Nigeria, I became a community nurse tutor in Brent Health District, with an office in the school of nursing at Central Middlesex Hospital. My role was to arrange in-service education for health visitors and district nurses and to teach student nurses about their work. It also included organising placements for the students with community nurses, as well as a day out with a public health inspector. Some students vowed never to eat in a restaurant again after witnessing cockroaches scurrying around the kitchens. Two friends who knew me from those days have recalled their impressions of me at the time.

Ursula said:

I had recently started my training at Central Middlesex Hospital and you had given us a lecture about going out into the community. My first impression at this point was of this young Black lady, with quite a huge afro, but you appeared extremely English. You were so conservatively dressed and I thought, oh dear. I didn't know you, obviously, as I didn't know there was a radical side to you.

Suzette said:

> We first met at Central Middlesex Hospital in the 1970s
> when I was working in the outpatient clinic and you
> were one of the tutors in the school of nursing. I was so
> taken aback because I had just finished my nurse training
> at Charing Cross and West London Hospital and now
> seeing someone Black at the School of Nursing was very,
> very unusual. It was inspirational for me. You were so
> enthusiastic, and I was really so surprised to see a Black
> woman in that position. What I observed is that you
> were sort of very English when you were at the School
> of Nursing. It was in your dress and in your approach
> to people. When you were in that school of nursing, it's
> like, you're a part of that white establishment. Yeah, but
> that all changed eventually.

Meanwhile, three things – which I call the three Ps: professional, personal and political – triggered me to get more
involved with sickle cell awareness and education. First was
my ignorance about the disease and my inability to be of
much help, when I was working as a health visitor in 1971,
to the devastated parents of children with the condition. I
always think of one little boy I met, who was around nine,
lying on his sofa, moaning in pain. Secondly, by now I had
a personal interest in the condition via my father. I'd been
introduced to a cousin called Nnamdi, who had sickle cell
anaemia. Joy's only living brother, he lived in Birmingham
and was to survive into his sixties. There had been a younger
sibling who had died in Nigeria and, while never diagnosed
with the illness, he had had a history of symptoms very
similar to Nnamdi's. Thirdly, being involved with the Black
community and Peter Moses' death in 1972 from leukaemia,

when Jessica had challenged my own lack of knowledge about sickle cell, had weighed heavily on my mind since.

It all came to a head in 1976 when I met Dr Milica Brozović, a consultant haematologist who had recently arrived at Central Middlesex Hospital. Known as Misha, she delivered two lunchtime talks about sickle cell disease and I made sure to attend both. They were inspiring and informative, but also made me angry that I had never been taught about the condition during my nursing or health visiting courses – both of which had taken place when London already had a significant African and Caribbean population. I wasn't alone in wondering whether the illness was so neglected because it mainly affects marginalised Black communities.

I remember asking Misha a lot of questions at each session. We had a discussion and she was delighted to learn of my strong community links – both as a specialist nurse tutor and through my involvement with Black voluntary groups. We hit it off straightaway and soon recognised our combined strengths in medical, nursing, teaching and community development. Our ambition was to raise the profile of the illness in order to improve care for patients, both within and outside of hospital. Our relationship was one of mutual respect and the recognition that, together, we could be a formidable team.

After her arrival at the hospital, Misha had been struck by how many patients were being admitted with excruciatingly painful sickle cell crises. What concerned her was the lack of knowledge about the illness among the patients, their families and the health professionals caring for them. In addition, the poor management of pain horrified her, as the staff didn't believe the severity of the pain, so when patients demanded medication, they would refuse to acknowledge the serious state of distress they were in. In 2016, a ground-breaking study entitled 'Racial bias in pain assessment and treatment recommendations, and false beliefs about biological differences between blacks and whites' detailed false beliefs of medical students and white laypeople, including 'Black people's skin is thicker than white people's skin'.[1]) It was an explosive mix of ignorance and racism from some of the staff. I will never forget how she described the scenes between some of the patients and staff as 'a battlefield'.

At a 1988 conference in Hackney, Misha recalled:

> Twelve years ago when I arrived at my present hospital, the Central Middlesex Hospital in Harlesden, I had never seen a patient with sickle cell disease. On my first day I was called: 'Dr B., could you come to ward D3 to deal with Francis?' 'Who is Francis?' 'Oh, he is a sickler.' 'What is wrong?' 'He is rolling on the floor, screaming at the top of his voice and using really unspeakable words.' 'Why is he doing it?' 'Oh, he is demanding pethidine.' 'Why is he demanding pethidine?' 'Because the nurses won't give him any more.'

Misha also observed that patients and the parents of children with sickle cell seemed very isolated and anxious. This reminded me of my health visiting days and the positive outcomes of bringing lonely mothers together at the toddler group. I offered to set up a support group with two interested local community nurses who had strong links with the hospital. Shirleen was a paediatric liaison health visitor and Cynthia a district nurse; both were of Caribbean origin and extremely keen.

After the second talk, back in 1976, Misha ran down the corridor after me and asked if I would be willing to see a

young adult on the male medical ward, as she was extremely
worried about him and the lack of concern from the nurses
and doctors. Yes, it was Francis, who Misha would later tell
people about in her talks. He was curled up in bed, facing
the wall and hidden under a blanket. I introduced myself
and explained my interest in sickle cell disease and that Dr
Brozović had asked me to visit him. After some time he turned
over, pulled his blanket down and stared at me for what seemed
an age. It was only when I mentioned our plans to set up a
support group that he became animated and interested, saying:
'I thought that I was the only person in Brent with sickle cell!'

Misha asked me to visit other patients, and one day I
went to the children's ward to see a teenage brother and
sister who were constantly being admitted. I let the office
know I was there and met their mother, who was delighted
to hear about the proposed group. During a subsequent visit
to see them, the sister told me about a very thin young girl
of about eight who had been admitted to their ward earlier
that day (being thin can be a classic sickle feature).

The two of them were concerned that the nurses didn't
appear to be taking any notice of the girl. She was under the
bedclothes quietly sobbing her little heart out and had been
in severe pain for many hours. I wasn't going to leave until
some pain relief had been administered, and I felt so much
anger. My professionalism kicked in, however; the nurses
knew me from around the hospital and my teaching, and I
politely but firmly suggested they administer some analgesic.
While I can be sympathetic to people not knowing about
the condition, this was in the late 1970s and the ward nurse
had a duty of care to these children.

The child's mother arrived and impressed upon me the fact
that unless she made a fuss, no one seemed to keep an eye on

her daughter. She was incredulous that some nurses claimed patients wanted medication to feed a drug addiction – even applying this argument in the case of a young child. It was an accusation that I was to hear time and time again, and from so many people. The mother was angry and frightened, but pleased when I offered to visit her at home. It soon became apparent that she'd received minimal information about the illness, and she eagerly soaked up what little I was able to provide.

Looking back, my refusal to be restricted by hospital and community boundaries was to be a key factor in breaking down barriers encountered by families. I was a guest in their homes, and it was often here that they revealed their fears, concerns and hopes for the future, and the stigma they were subjected to. The hospital nursing staff appreciated my growing knowledge of the illness and positive rapport with patients, some of whom they viewed as 'difficult'. Possible reasons for the latter are to be found in the excellent and controversial 1972 publication *The Unpopular Patient* by nurse researcher Dr Felicity Stockwell, in which she draws out how some nurses considered people who challenged their control to be 'awkward customers'.

Throughout this period, my thirst for travel never abated, helped enormously by the introduction of much lower airfares through so-called bucket shops and Freddie Laker's cheap transatlantic flights. I visited several countries for the first time, including Morocco. In the summer of 1976, I stayed at the Nigerian Embassy in Rabat with my diplomat uncle Akudo and his young family. He helped towards the cost of the air ticket as a present for having chauffeured him around London the previous year.

Six months following this trip, I would formally change my surname to Anionwu. I had thought long and hard about the pros and cons of continuing to use my mother's maiden name versus switching to my father's surname. One decisive factor was the visit to Nigeria, as well as socialising with the Igbo community in London. When I was in Onitsha, Anionwu rather than Furlong was used – for example, when relatives purchased my internal airline tickets. One cousin joked that I was a typical *oyinbo* to worry about whether officials would notice the different name on my passport.

It amused me that in England there may well have been in-depth discussions about this before reaching a decision, whereas in Nigeria it seemed ridiculous even to raise the subject. 'You are the daughter of Anionwu, what is the problem?' Well, I had spent twenty-nine years of my life known to the world as Furlong. How would my mother and members of my maternal family react when I informed them about this change in name? What of all those people I knew professionally and socially? There was also the rigmarole of having to change all of my official records and inform so many agencies, which at times appeared quite daunting. My mind was eventually made up, though, and so on 12 July 1976 I changed my surname to Anionwu by deed poll. There was no negative response from my mother, and, knowing her, I have a feeling she would have been quietly pleased.

The impact was interesting, because I had switched to a name that many people found much more difficult to pronounce, including me. My anglicised phonetic version, 'Annie-on-woo', wasn't exactly as Igbo people would say it, but better than the experience of being called Elizabeth Onion. This was an introduction to the difficulties I would face in the future. When I was on the phone and told people my surname, there was sometimes a noticeable difference in reactions. Before, having a non-foreign-sounding name and a very English accent, people were totally unaware of my skin colour. Occasionally, there would even be attempts to encourage me to collude with their racist comments. No longer, thank goodness, due to my now decidedly 'alien-sounding' name. On 18 August 1976, I obtained a new passport in the name of Anionwu.

Chapter 32:

The First UK Sickle Cell Nurse

Volunteering with Misha, we took a two-pronged approach to address the key issues of educating health professionals about sickle cell and providing support for patients and families. The first was to organise a sickle cell seminar in February that was attended by over 200 hospital and community health staff. During the planning stages, I came across a brief reference in a medical journal journal about the launch in May 1976 of OSCAR, the Organisation for Sickle Cell Anaemia Research, which was a national organisation tackling sickle cell awareness and support. We invited Neville Clare, a co-founder who had sickle cell disease, to give a talk.

Secondly, and a month later, our local support group held their inaugural meeting, and my community links were to prove very helpful. We obtained, free of charge, a room at the Learie Constantine Centre, which was a community venue often used by local Caribbean groups. Contacts within the Black media also resulted in welcome publicity, including a radio interview on Alex Pascall's pioneering BBC Radio *Black Londoners* programme. The *West Indian World* newspaper also included a free advert about the event. As a result, sixteen people attended, as well as Shirleen, Cynthia and myself, and we were all very heartened by the enthusiasm.

Misha encouraged me to write up the outcome, and this became my first-ever publication about sickle cell disease. Called 'Self-Help in Sickle Cell Anaemia', it was published on 21 September 1977 in *World Medicine* magazine. Nowadays, support groups are common for many health conditions, but rereading the article reminded me how unique it was back then, certainly for sickle cell disease:

> The people attending ranged from a mother with her three children (she had lost a sixteen-year-old daughter last year following a cerebrovascular accident during a crisis) to a cheerful twenty-year-old who arrived by motorbike – and contrasted sharply with a twenty-six-year-old man who was ill and depressed, having entered hospital six times during the past year. It was the first opportunity for almost all of them to meet anyone else with the same condition. The effect was dramatic: one could feel the sense of relief they experienced; and the surprise to find they were not alone was clear on their faces.

The group was called Brent OSCAR and met regularly. They also raised funds to produce education materials and buy a film projector, essential for the frequent talks and film shows now being organised. Previously stigmatised individuals and families were becoming more confident about speaking to journalists and opening up about the impact of the illness.

By now, I'd also realised the need to study for a degree in order to progress to an even more senior level, and obtained a place on a two-year master's degree in Tropical Health at the Liverpool School of Tropical Medicine, due to start in the autumn of 1976. I was also awarded, for two years, the very first King's Fund scholarship, which had been established to assist senior nurses to obtain a higher degree and undertake research.

All was going swimmingly until the 1976 programme in Liverpool was suddenly cancelled and, consequently, I was unable to take up the scholarship. Bitterly disappointed, I looked around for a different course and, in 1977, accepted an offer from the Department of Nursing at the University of Manchester. The plan was to complete a two-year programme – first the advanced diploma, followed by an MSc in nursing studies. Fortunately, the King's Fund again agreed to give me the scholarship and one of my key supporters was Robert J. Maxwell, their secretary and chief executive.

The first year of study in Manchester put me off the idea of continuing to complete the master's degree. The overall philosophy appeared to be focused narrowly on the nursing process, a theory of nursing practice very fashionable at the time. It was too hospital-centred for my liking and not flexible enough even to incorporate a community-based placement. Nor was there much enthusiasm for my wish to do a dissertation on sickle cell disease. The local Clinical Genetics Unit were friendly but admitted that they rarely received referrals to provide genetic counselling for affected families. Apart from the odd general practitioner, there was no alternative provision within the community, as I discovered through my links with Black community groups in Manchester.

An idea came to me as to how I could adapt the nursing process in order to incorporate a more home-based perspective. I organised a placement on the children's infectious diseases ward at Wythenshawe Hospital, assuming that most of the patients would have a short admission. This turned out to be the case, and I was able to obtain consent from parents to visit them both on the ward and at home. My interviews with the parents explored the impact of the inpatient experience and the transition home following the child's discharge from hospital.

My frustration with the nursing course was balanced with an exciting time in Manchester and making friends with students on other courses when I joined the university's Pan-African Student Association. There, I met two wonderful women – Duduzile Lethlaku from the former Bophuthat-swana (now part of South Africa), and Olive Morris, the now deceased Brixton-based community activist who set up the Brixton Black Women's group in 1973 and became an influential Black feminist and activist before her untimely death at the age of twenty-seven from non-Hodgkin lymphoma.

We three 'Amazonians' gave some of the more misogynistic men in the Pan-African Student Association a run for their money, helping to block moves to exclude women from positions of influence and decision-making processes. Life became much more interesting, as I spent time volunteering at the Black Women's Co-operative in Moss Side. The three of us also used to travel down to London regularly in my Mini for meetings of the newly formed OWAAD (Organisation of Women of African and Asian Descent), which has since been described as 'a watershed in the history of Black women's rights activism',[1] campaigning against increased immigration restrictions and deportation, domestic violence, children's exclusion from schools, policing, health and reproductive rights.

In 1977, Dad stayed with me for a few days in the flat I was sharing in London. At some point during his visit he asked why I hadn't bought my own place instead of wasting money on renting. My immediate reply was that while my salary was sufficient for the monthly mortgage repayments, I didn't have the money for a deposit. He gave me useful advice about always saving a percentage of my monthly earnings. Then, to my surprise, he offered to give me the deposit on a flat as well as paying the legal fees. The only requirement was that the property should be accessible from Heathrow Airport so he could stay with me when he was in London.

In July 1978, having completed the advanced diploma at the University of Manchester, I returned to London with the hope of finding an MSc degree in health education. The person I spoke to at the Health Education Council pointed out that even if I obtained a place at this late stage, there still remained the challenge of meeting the course fees. He was quite taken aback when I told him of my remaining year of the King's Fund scholarship and suggested contacting the health education guru Alan Beattie. When I met Alan, he had recently been appointed director of the MSc in health education programme at Chelsea College, University of London. He said: 'You immediately struck me as vigorous, energetic, animated, passionate, showing a real professional and practical concern about the issue of sickle cell disease, and, from what you told me, the situation for families was rather horrifying.'

After a long discussion, we decided that the ideal plan would be for me to undertake a research-based MPhil degree rather than the two-year part-time taught master's course. The problem was that, even with my recent Manchester qualification, I didn't meet the academic requirements to register for a University of London postgraduate degree. Alan worked incredibly hard on my behalf, together with his head of department and university administrators. It was agreed that I could register, with the requirement that I sit (as qualifying examinations) the most pertinent papers from the MSc in health education – epidemiology and research methods.

So, over the next two years I sat in on relevant sections of the course in preparation for the exams. Following my return to London, Dr Brozović had also appointed me as Research Fellow in her haematology department. By now I had become more interested in putting my energies into developing services for families affected by sickle cell disease in the UK. While still enjoying trips to Nigeria, my vision of working there had started to fade.

My first project with Misha was to develop a register of local patients. Using hospital activity analysis data, all records were pulled that included the diagnostic code for sickle cell disease. I stayed on at work for many a long evening ploughing through hospital medical notes. A total of fifty-seven patients with sickle cell disease were identified, and numerous errors discovered in the other records. Blood results neatly pasted in the notes revealed these individuals to have sickle cell trait and *not* sickle cell disease. It was yet another illustration of the utter confusion there was between sickle cell trait and the illness itself. I also came across a lack of knowledge about the Caribbean and where many of the patients came from, as exemplified by one doctor writing: 'I examined this pleasant Jamaican lady from Barbados . . .'

(In January 1981, our article describing the characteristics of seventy patients was published in the prestigious *British Medical Journal*. Entitled 'Sickle Cell Disease in a British Urban Community', the paper was produced by a team of us that included Misha, Dr Diana Walford, both haematologists, and a statistician, Dr Betty Kirkwood. It was the first paper of its kind in the UK, and I was pleasantly surprised when Misha made me first author. It was so typical of the way she acknowledged my contribution, even though I wasn't a medical doctor and had only recently commenced work on my MPhil, which I went on to convert to a PhD – pretty unusual for someone who left school at sixteen. Later on in my academic career, I became aware that this wasn't always standard practice; Misha also taught me about the power of disseminating evidence through mainstream professional journals.)

The pilot study for my PhD degree entailed interviewing five parents from outside Brent. The account of one mother formed the basis of an article in *Nursing Times* in July 1979. Called 'Learning to Cope with Sickle Cell Disease – A Parent's Experience', it was written in collaboration with my supervisor Alan Beattie. 'Miss J', as I called the mother, had been identified as having sickle cell trait during pregnancy but wasn't informed of this until just before she had her son. Following his birth, she asked two different doctors if her son would get the illness and each said, no, he would be fine. His first admission to hospital at ten months of age lasted four weeks, and that was when he was diagnosed with sickle cell anaemia. She told me: 'I don't know whether I was coming or going. I thought I would die, actually, because I was walking like I'm not walking at all. I think I was floating, and every time, every day I went up to see him, he looked like he was finished.' Many parents spoke about their dreadful experiences, mirroring those of Miss J. Only one woman had ever heard of sickle cell at the time of diagnosis (in a child whom she and her husband had adopted). All of the mothers had been identified as carriers during pregnancy, but none had been informed of their result and no partners were offered screening. No baby was tested at birth, even though it was possible to do so. The relevant investigation, haemoglobin electrophoresis, had been developed during the 1950s and wasn't expensive. It amazed me that screening and clinical care for sickle cell disease had such a low priority, given that it was one of the first conditions to be recognised as a molecular disease.

My main study involved interviewing twenty-two parents of children with sickle cell disease who had been followed at Central Middlesex Hospital from 1962 onwards. My mother very kindly transcribed all the recorded interviews, which lasted forty to ninety minutes, for which I was immensely grateful. We would have conversations about the research, as I was primarily interviewing mothers and fathers from Caribbean and African origin, so some of them had strong accents or used a little bit of slang. My mother would call and say, 'I'm not sure I've got this word,' and I'd explain it to her. She found the content very interesting, and it gave her a much better insight into what I was doing, so we'd talk about that.

My increasing involvement with sickle cell made me realise that the US was the best place to visit in view of the developments that had occurred there since 1972. So, in August 1977, I decided to go on holiday to Los Angeles, staying with my cousin Obiageli and her family. While there, I could also undertake a sickle cell fact-finding mission. In addition, I discovered that the National Association for Sickle Cell Disease (now the Sickle Cell Disease Association of America) and a local group were located in the same city. Both generously donated leaflets, posters and films for me to take back to London. They advised me to return in September of the following year, during National Sickle Cell Awareness Month, and invited me to speak at their Annual General Meeting and conference in Minneapolis.

At the conference, I met delegates from all over the country. As happened during my first trip in 1971, many thought I was an African-American due to my huge afro hairstyle and they were always pleasantly surprised to hear my English accent. For example, my British pronunciation of the word 'capillary' was quite different from the US version. They were also astonished to hear about the significant Black and minority ethnic presence in the UK and that sickle cell disease was an issue.

During my visit, the national organisation generously arranged for me to attend an intensive haemoglobinopathy counselling course at the Oakland's Children's Hospital Medical Center of Northern California. It covered sickle cell and thalassaemia, the latter being a severe inherited anaemia requiring monthly blood transfusions. The course provided me with a wonderful opportunity to get to know the delegates, mainly African-American nurses. Their generosity was overwhelming. We all got on incredibly well, and they virtually adopted me for the week.

In the US, nationally funded comprehensive sickle cell centres were created through funds generated following the 1972 National Sickle Cell Disease Control Act. This legislation arose from lobbying by sickle cell groups, health specialists, the Black Panther Party and the media. A significant amount of credit is also given to Colby King, a Black research fellow at the Department of Health, Education and Welfare (HEW), who would later win the 2003 Pulitzer Prize for Commentary.

In the autumn of 1970, King was assigned to prepare a report about the response of the National Institutes of Health (NIH) to sickle cell. The project had been prompted by a letter from the mother of an affected child writing to the department, asking for help. King demonstrated NIH's low priority and minimal resources allocated to sickle cell disease in comparison to funds approved for conditions of equal or lesser prevalence. He also identified the lack of equitable representation on NIH advisory boards, with only one Black member out of 113.[2]

His report was submitted to Robert Patricelli, a deputy undersecretary at HEW at a time when officials were preparing options for President Nixon's Health Message. Patricelli also discussed the report with his father, Leonard, who was President of WITC, a Connecticut television station. The latter decided that his station would run a campaign 'to do something about sickle cell anemia.' He kept his word, and November 1970 saw the launch of the first detailed and influential TV and radio series on sickle cell disease. By April 1971, they had raised nearly $34,000 to establish the first comprehensive paediatric sickle cell centre at Washington DC's Howard University. This was prior to the national government funds released following the rapidly written and enacted 1972 National Sickle Cell Disease Control Act.[3] (There would be some parallels in England thirty years later, with the last-minute inclusion of a funded screening programme for sickle and thalassaemia in the ten-year NHS Plan, launched in 2000.[4])

All of these US activities coincided with the aftermath of the civil rights movement. The title of the Act highlights the apparently contentious objective of reducing the number of cases through screening populations for sickle cell trait. There was a huge outcry, as this was perceived to be a eugenic measure against predominantly Black at-risk communities. So there was a major effort to clarify that funding was for comprehensive centres to deliver care and undertake research, as well as screening and genetic counselling.

By 1976, there were fifteen such centres, and I visited the San Francisco centre, where I spent time with Sylvia

Lee, an African-American paediatric nurse practitioner, who had seven years' experience in sickle cell disease. Her philosophy of care influenced me immensely and gave me the opportunity to see a Black nurse working in this way. It gave me the idea that once back in Brent I, too, could develop a similar service.

In my report of this mind-blowing trip, I observed:

It is apparent that great strides have been achieved in the United States in the last seven years or so, but that this is perhaps just the start of a realisation that sickle cell disease must now be treated as a major health problem for some foreseeable time. There are many lessons to be learned from the American experience for the situation that exists in Britain, as it is in a similar position the USA found itself during the period of the late sixties and early seventies. That is, sickle cell disease is a low health priority with no health education material, very little awareness among both the professional and lay community, and virtually no specialised support for affected individuals and families.

In September 1979, Misha obtained two rooms at Willesden Hospital. From here, I ran the Brent Sickle Cell and Thalassaemia Information, Screening and Counselling Centre. It was the first such service of its type in the UK, making me the country's very first sickle cell and thalassaemia nurse specialist; I would remain the only one here for six years.

From the outset, Misha and I decided that we needed to obtain resources to develop awareness programmes for lay and professional groups. The lack of knowledge concerning the true prevalence of sickle cell also needed to be addressed. It was clear from the patients we had met that there was an urgent requirement for specialist medical care, information and support. Moreover, a few years previously, I had come across this astonishing statement in a 1976 book entitled *Genetic Counselling* by Alan Stevenson and Clare Davison: 'Sickle-cell anaemia is not of great consequence to us in the context of genetic counselling in the United Kingdom. The sickling trait and sickle cell anaemia appear to be confined to peoples of African and Eastern origin.' This shocking ignorance was a key driver that led me to travel all the way to the US to access training in sickle cell and thalassaemia genetic counselling.

An open-door blood testing facility was vital to reduce the barriers for those wishing to know their haemoglobin type. Fortunately, blood samples could be taken at the hospital. Misha arranged for people to access this service without the need for a referral from a family doctor. I was authorised to complete the relevant blood investigation request forms. This all seemed quite revolutionary in those days.

I ran the genetic counselling sessions and arranged family studies. Misha and I had previously visited our local regional clinical genetics centre to establish what services they provided. We were given a very warm reception but, while there was genetic counselling for cystic fibrosis, there were no similar services for sickle cell and thalassaemia apart from the very occasional referral. There was an incorrect assumption that general practitioners, paediatricians and haematologists were addressing these needs. No effort seemed to have been made to establish whether this was actually the case.

I was also fortunate to be awarded a fellowship to study sickle cell service from the Commission for Racial Equality (CRE) in 1979, which enabled me to visit the Caribbean countries of Jamaica, Barbados, Trinidad and Tobago, St Lucia and also Guyana in South America. These fantastic opportunities provided me with so many insights that were to be of great help in developing services in Brent, learning about services for marginalised communities and attitudes and health beliefs towards sickle cell disorders.

During my stay in Guyana in July 1979, I reconnected with my old friend Walter Rodney, who I'd first met through his publisher. He was still a major political activist and not at all popular with the government in power. Our meeting was organised in great secrecy due to the many death threats he had received. A car arrived to take me to his current address – he moved homes frequently – and a few minutes into the journey I was taken aback to hear Rodney's voice: he was hidden under a blanket in the back of the car.

He told me all about the current political tensions and the numerous street demonstrations that he'd spoken at. I told him about my own experience the previous day, when I was arrested in the street for taking photographs in the capital of Georgetown. The policeman informed me that my camera had been aimed at the headquarters of the People's National Congress (PNC), the political party that was in power. He refused to believe that I was actually taking a photo of a beautiful Hindu temple.

A crowd gathered and they soon elicited the fact that I was from London and that my trip was concerned with sickle cell. They all rounded on the policeman and formed a barrier between us, at which point somebody gave me a lift back to where I was staying. As in 1970 in Paris, my hobby of photography had once again got me into trouble. Sadly, this would be the last time I would see Rodney, as he was assassinated in Guyana the following year, on 13 June 1980, and just one day after my father's death.

Chapter 33:

Losing My Father

Although it started off well, with a couple of cheerful letters from my father, 1980 was to be a very shocking year. On 9 January, he wrote of his plans to come to London for ten days, following a visit to Los Angeles to see Emma, who was at university there, and Obiageli. He seemed fine when he arrived to stay with me in February.

On my return from a few days away, Dad greeted me in the hall and started to apologise for having broken a glass and for spilling water on the carpet. I quickly saw that all was not well with him physically. He seemed to have had a stroke – his speech was slightly slurred and his face was drooping on one side. I asked him how he was feeling and whether he had any weakness down one side of his body, and he said, yes, looking at me in a very scared manner. I immediately drove him to the accident and emergency unit of Central Middlesex Hospital. It did indeed turn out that he had had a mild stroke, which was a great shock to everyone. He was advised to lose weight, cut down on smoking and flying, and was prescribed medication to reduce his blood pressure. It was very reassuring that he was in a hospital where I knew so many nurses and doctors.

Dad, ever the diplomat, proved to be an extremely popular patient. So much so that he managed to persuade a nurse to buy him chocolate, which he was thoroughly enjoying one day when I visited him. The nurse in question said that it was impossible to refuse, as he was such a polite, charming and humorous patient. When my father joked and said he wasn't feeling ill, it dawned on me that he didn't appreciate the serious nature of his illness. I explained the dangers of another stroke and he asked me whether it could kill him. It hurt me so much to reply in the affirmative and see the look of shock on his face.

When he was well enough, Dad returned to Nigeria, and the plan was that I would visit him in the summer. A month later, he wrote to give me an update on his health. Dated 15 April, his letter informed me that his blood pressure was well down and his weight had also been decreasing (it was now steady at fourteen and a half stone). Nonetheless, it was a surprise to receive a phone call in June from my father and to hear that he was now in the US. He had felt well enough to travel to Chicago to attend the Rotary International Convention, accompanied by his good friend Mr Albert Osakwe. He'd also seen Emma graduate from his university in LA and was about to come and spend a few days with me in London, then return to Nigeria. I was anxious about the impact of all this international travel so soon after his stroke.

When my father arrived at Heathrow Airport on Monday, 9 June 1980, he telephoned to let me know that he would come by Tube to the flat. His voice sounded so tired that I said, 'Look, Dad, just wait and I'll come and meet you at the airport.' My fears about his health were confirmed when I saw the look of utter exhaustion on his face as he pushed his luggage trolley towards me. I suggested that he rest as much as possible for the next few days prior to his flight back to

Nigeria. He agreed to do this but asked if I could arrange an appointment with a solicitor and requested that I come with him. He wished to discuss the property in Palmers Green, as he and Regi were now on such bad terms that he was considering a divorce.

We went to the solicitors on the Tuesday. When he was called in, I remained seated, but he turned and beckoned for me to come with him. As a result, I heard his anxieties about the marriage and his wish for the house to be transferred from joint ownership to his name alone. On the final night of his stay, we had a meal together and then both retired to bed early. He was due to fly out to Nigeria the next morning and I was going to drive him to the airport.

On waking that morning of Thursday, 12 June 1980, I could hear a slight grunting noise from the bathroom. There was no reply when I knocked on the door, so I opened it and to my absolute horror I found my father unconscious in the bath. I called an ambulance and he was taken once more to Central Middlesex Hospital. It was clear that his condition was extremely serious. The doctors prepared me for the worst. I sat by his bed for most of that day, intermittently making phone calls to inform relatives and friends. A few were able to come and visit him, and they gave me tremendous support, as did the hospital staff. One of the nurses I knew even arranged for me to have a quick shower. My father was deeply unconscious and at one point a young female doctor told me that he was rapidly deteriorating. I kissed him goodbye, and very soon after that he was pronounced dead.

Mr Osakwe, who had so recently been in Chicago with my father, fainted when his son phoned him in Nigeria to tell him the news. At some point later, it struck me that three days after my father's death had marked the eighth anniversary of our first meeting on 15 June 1972. His death certificate stated his age as fifty-nine. Whether this was his actual age, or whether he was in fact sixty-two (as suggested by his old Cambridge college records that I tracked down in 2013), he was still young when he died.

My world seemed to come crashing down around me. The day after my father's death was when Jessica told me that Rodney had been assassinated. She knew my dad had died, so she said over the phone, 'I'm really sorry, girl, but Walter has been murdered.' We knew the threats were there, so it didn't come as a massive surprise, but it did come as a big shock.

Fortunately, friends, family and associates of my father provided me with constant support. My mother wrote: 'I was very sorry to hear about your dad. I can well imagine how upset you must be. Try not to grieve too much. It's the last thing he would wish.'

My distress wasn't eased by Emma, who was due to stay with me on his return from Los Angeles. My keenness to help him at our time of bereavement quickly diminished due to his arrogant and selfish behaviour. He had hardly set foot in the hallway when he demanded papers for my flat, assuming it was now in his possession (a couple of years later, in 1982, during the period when Regi and Emma were still at loggerheads about Dad's estate, she wrote to me: 'For your amusement, your flat belongs to Emmanuel too!').

Tired and stressed out with it all, I lost my temper with Emma and rang my cousins to share what had happened. They immediately came to collect him and gave him a unique Nigerian dressing-down, physically scooping him up, making it very clear that they were furious with him.

This flash of greed was to be a mere taste of what I would come to experience.

At this time, I was revising for an exam at the Institute of Education that would enable me to register for my MPhil. Interventions were made on my behalf and I was allowed to delay the exam until I had returned home from my father's funeral, which was to be held in Nigeria.

The whole period of organising for his body to be taken back to Nigeria was hazy, as is a lot of the period leading up to the burial. The Nigerian government, their officials in London and my father's friends saw to everything. Due to his previous roles as the first Permanent Secretary of the Ministry of External Affairs, then Nigerian Ambassador to Italy, officialdom stepped in and everything was fast-tracked. When my Anionwu relatives and I landed at the airport in Lagos on 18 June, we were met on the tarmac and driven off at speed with a police escort all the way to Onitsha. This, my father's last journey home, was in stark contrast to that first car trip together in 1973.

During the ten days before the funeral, rumours flew about the possible causes of his death, including poisoning. Emma stated that Dad's enemies had invoked evil spirits to kill him, as during the night he'd heard three cocks crowing on the roof of the house. Being the last person to see him alive, I was bombarded with questions and conspiracy theories until members of the family intervened on my behalf.

One day I was in the sitting room of my father's house with family members receiving condolences from visitors. A wailing sound was suddenly heard, which got louder and louder until a distressed woman made a dramatic entrance. Approaching me, she prostrated herself on the floor, sobbing something in Igbo. A relative informed me that she was the mother of three of Dad's children, the half-siblings my father had introduced me to on a previous visit. All this sounds both gloomy and frightening, but it was tempered with overwhelming comfort from a wide range of people – and while at Onitsha, I came to realise that Nigerian wakes are very similar to those of the Irish. Stories were recalled about my father and many jokes were told about him, which I found incredibly therapeutic.

Several obituary notices appeared in the Nigerian media posted by family and friends, as well as one in the *Daily Star* on 26 June 1980 from the Onitsha branch of the Nigerian Bar Association, of which my father was Chairman. *West Africa* magazine also included an obituary to him.

The burial service took place at All Saints Cathedral, Onitsha, on Saturday, 28 June 1980, and photos taken at the service show me looking absolutely distraught. My father's peers from the local branch of the Nigerian Bar Association, all wearing their legal robes and wigs, carried the coffin into the cathedral. They also processed with the coffin to the burial plot within the grounds of his house in his beloved village of Ogboli Eke.

An unsuccessful search for my father's will commenced in London, Lagos and Onitsha. The latter produced a moment of dark humour as I accompanied a group of people hunting through papers at his office. Mr Osakwe pulled me to one side and asked me to distract an elder, as they had come across that gentleman's last will and testament and weren't keen for him to know they had seen it.

On my return to Heathrow Airport, a great friend of my father, Chief Rex Edijana Akpofure, met me on the tarmac. He had been the first African principal of Dad's alma mater, King's College, Lagos. I stayed with his family and he then accompanied me to the Institute of Education, where I was to sit my postponed exam, and into a vast hall, empty bar one invigilator. Alan Beattie recalled: 'You sat [your exams] after everybody else but under rigorous examination conditions, policed and invigilated to boot. You duly passed.' A few days later on 2 July (my thirty-third birthday), a photo of me at Chief Akpofure's home shows me smiling and looking much more relaxed.

The next few years were to prove extremely difficult, particularly in terms of my relationship with my stepmother, Regi, and my brother Emma. It soon transpired that my father, although a barrister, hadn't left a will and therefore died intestate. The wrangling about his estate would carry on for decades, although after a few years I dropped out of the whole vicious affair. It is still painful to recall the spiteful intensity with which certain parties looked after their own interests while colluding to exclude others, including myself.

There was no love lost between Regi and Emma as they battled their counterclaims out in the courts. Regi wrote frequent letters asking me for my signature on various documents and constantly complaining about Emma's behaviour. This included how, with a forged letter, he had closed his father's bank account in Los Angeles after withdrawing all the funds. These, she continued in a letter dated 13 January 1982, were spent on a car that was later sold, and flights around America and Italy: 'Really he cannot be a son of your dad.'

Advised to seek legal redress, for a few years I hired an Onitsha-based lawyer recommended by the family. As the years passed, it struck me that I was wasting what little money was in my bank account. Emma had now sided with my stepmother and I eventually decided not to pursue any further action.

I realised that the only important thing was the joy of having known my father for eight years, and that we had got on extremely well. I was really lucky to have had the good fortune to find him so quickly, in contrast to those who had failed in their efforts to trace their biological parent or patents. I'd been introduced to many positive aspects of Nigerian family life and culture. My father had advised me so well about my career and had also given me funds to secure a mortgage. I reflected, though, that property and money weren't anything if you didn't also have a decent family life and a wonderful network of friends.

After my father's funeral, members of the Anionwu family pleaded with me to come back soon, as they were afraid that I would never return. As a result, my next trip was just seven months later in December 1980. I stayed with my father's friends, the Mbanefo family, due to the severe tensions with Regi concerning the estate. Once back in London, I realised I wasn't sure when I would return, as it would never be the same without Dad.

There was no doubt that I fell in love with Nigeria from my very first visit in 1973. Like a pendulum, my cultural loyalties shifted, so much so that I initially wanted to emigrate. Although those rose-tinted glasses did eventually fade a little, and while I ultimately never settled there, I was to make many more trips in the future. I still feel a huge affection for and interest in the affairs of the country and take the greatest pride in the origins of my father.

Chapter 34:

A New Road

Meeting my father had rounded off my whole being and filled in those many gaps concerning my identity. It also increased my self-confidence, as evidenced by my taking on his surname while retaining pride in my mother's heritage. Taking this decision had been unexpectedly liberating, as I had at last defined myself. This was in defiance of having an identity externally foisted on me by those wishing to label me by the colour of my skin, with all the associated negative assumptions. As Elizabeth Nneka Anionwu, I would go into the next phase of life helped by names that reflected my entire roots. As a Black woman, I'd gained confidence to campaign with others and make a real change.

Since its creation in 1977, our local group, Brent OSCAR, had gained significant publicity and an increased profile, soon becoming better known than the national OSCAR group. This caused so many tensions that eventually our local group decided unanimously to break away and in 1979 adopted a new name: the Sickle Cell Society. Funds were raised for national dissemination of information, a welfare fund, scholarships and an annual children's holiday. The society also supported local health services – purchasing a computer for the Brent Centre and laboratory equipment to screen newborn babies at Central Middlesex Hospital.

I also acted as a voluntary information officer for the society. At the time, the official estimate was that at least 3,000 people in Britain were affected by sickle cell – which was disputed by the charity as a gross underestimate. Campaigning became a critical part of our work, with one of the best examples being the October 1981 report *Sickle Cell Disease: The Need for Improved Services*. This highlighted the difficulties faced by families up and down the country, using information gleaned from letters and phone calls to the society, as well as input at public meetings. In 1991, a third edition of this report was published, and it noted that in 1986 there was an estimated 5,000 cases of sickle cell disease. The report contained twenty-four recommendations for improving services, including the need for a national policy to screen babies, the collection of statistics about incidence and death rates, and guidelines for casualty and inpatient care, together with follow-up at specialist clinics.

The pioneering NHS service that Misha and I had set up in Brent also created huge interest both in the country and the media. Membership of the Sickle Cell Society charity grew at a rapid rate and celebrity patrons were appointed, such as comedian (now Sir) Lenny Henry and children's television presenter (now Baroness) Floella Benjamin. There were interviews and numerous talks given at public meetings, and money was raised to produce information. In 1983, the Sickle Cell Society obtained funding from Thames Television Telethon for a long-overdue publication, *A Handbook on Sickle Cell Disease: A Guide for Families*, which I wrote with June Hall, a teacher and trustee of the charity. It was illustrated by Bryan Jones, a young artist affected by sickle cell anaemia, who sadly died a few years later.

An immensely gratifying venture was the regular specialist one-week courses that Misha and I organised from the Brent

Centre. These were partially driven by my own experience of having to travel all the way to the US to study but were also in response to numerous requests for training from health professionals and voluntary groups up and down the country. An example comes from Alison, a former clinical scientist laboratory director in Cardiff:

> I phoned up Brent Sickle Cell Centre out of desperation to find information for somebody in the community venturing into doing something to fill the gap in services. That person had watched a feature on [the television programme] Black on Black. We were absolutely dependent on the generosity of people, and being part of that growing national network of nurse counsellors and community initiatives.

In spring 1981, I was awarded a Churchill Fellowship to travel to five cities in the US and to undertake a one-month visit to Jamaica as a fact-finding opportunity. While visiting Washington DC, I stayed with Sarah, my friend from my Paris days, who had now returned to the US. It was while I was there that on 30 March 1981, just down the street from her house, there was an assassination attempt on President Ronald Reagan. Watching the endless replays on television, I suddenly heard a man calling my name from downstairs. Peering over the bannister and seeing guns pointed at me, I just froze in fear. As Sarah recounted: 'You had left the downstairs door ajar, and I had called the police, having recently had a robbery, [but I had] also let them know you were staying with me. The lights weren't on, and it was dusk. All you could see were two crouching male figures, with guns drawn!'

This was not the best timing, as I had recently found out I was pregnant. In January 1981, I'd gone to the wedding of my Nigerian friend Kezi and met Nick. He was the best friend of the groom and was studying for a PhD in chemistry at a Yorkshire university. While born in Northern Nigeria, he was an Igbo from a village near Onitsha (as a teenager, his father had been killed during the massacres of Igbos in the north that led to the Biafra War). We hit it off straightaway and were on the dance floor together for most of the night.

Over the next three months, we met up a lot, enjoying each other's company. Everything seemed on track for us to have a future together and we both felt it was the right time for us to have a child. My father's death, nine months earlier, had triggered an instinctive desire to start my own family. Now aged thirty-four, my body clock had begun to tick; Nick was only a month younger than me.

I thought, a little naively, that even if we split up it would be possible for me to cope with being a single mother. I had a flat, a job and a great network of close friends, including Dolores, a childminder with whom I had become friends during my days as a health visitor. She always said that she would look after any children I might have, and I had every intention of taking her up on it.

When I became pregnant so quickly, it was an eye-opener to witness the reaction of family, friends and colleagues. Some thought I was too bookish and work-driven ever to imagine that a child would feature in my life. Others were amazed, as I had never spoken to them about my private life, leading them to presume that men didn't feature in it. The most interesting response was the manner in which a few people from Onitsha probed the identity of the soon-to-be father.

They smiled and uttered a satisfied '*Eh-he!*' whenever they were pleased with my response during their interrogation:

'Is he Black?'

'Yes.'

'West Indian?'

'No.'

'Nigerian?'

'Yes.'

'Igbo?'

'Yes.'

The excitement was mounting.

'Is he from Onitsha?'

'No.'

They looked quite disappointed until one of them said, 'Oh well, you tried!', to which they all agreed while beaming at me.

Motherhood was an important rite of passage in their eyes so, regardless of my single status, they were genuinely thrilled with the news. When I told Sarah during my trip to Washington, she insisted, in her wonderfully forthright way, that I mustn't drink any coffee or alcohol for the rest of the pregnancy. (And so it was, but pretty soon after the baby was born, I asked for a very strong coffee. In contrast, I never missed alcohol and it wasn't until the christening that I supped some champagne. The taste was so awful that I became teetotal.)

There was never a hint of morning sickness in those early months, which was fortunate in view of the amount of air travel involved in touring five US cities and then on to Jamaica. By 11 May, I was at the laboratories of the Medical Research Council Sickle Cell Unit in Kingston. The radio was on and suddenly someone shouted that Bob Marley had died in Miami. Nine days later, courtesy of a nurse from the unit who had sweet-talked a policeman, we managed to jump the queue and see the singer lying in state at Kingston's National Arena.

I also took the test confirming my pregnancy in this laboratory. Apart from severe heartburn in the later stages, I would find pregnancy was wonderful. My weight did balloon though, due to a craving for buttered toast and milk. On the plus side, my skin tone improved and my hair became even curlier. It's interesting that I cannot recall the moment I told my mother, or her reaction, but she never expressed any signs of shock or disapproval.

Chapter 35:

Single Motherhood

My friend Janet asked me to call her as soon as regular contractions started in December, as she wanted to be with me for the delivery as Nick was up in Yorkshire. It happened to be one of the coldest months in years when my labour kicked off, and snow was heavy on the ground as she drove me to the hospital. I was supposed to have a 'trial of labour', which meant that a caesarean section would be performed if no progress was made within a short period of time. This was because my hips were assessed as bordering on being too narrow, which might result in the baby getting stuck. That's exactly what happened, and after many hours there were signs that my unborn baby was in distress.

It was all very frightening and made worse on overhearing that the anaesthetist couldn't be found. Hours elapsed and the pain was becoming unbearable. The agony wasn't due to contractions but horrendous pain in my right lower back, later pinpointed to the sacroiliac joint. An epidural eventually relieved the agony, but labour lasted for a total of twenty-two hours. All this time Janet had been wonderful, but she needed to go home to her own children. Fortunately, my friend Cynthia took over; she was also pregnant, and I worried about the impact this complicated labour might have on her. A decision was eventually taken to deliver the baby by Kielland's forceps. It was now evening, and by this stage I was convinced that the baby couldn't possibly survive and was preparing for the worst.

All was well, though, and my healthy baby came screaming into the world at last. I immediately burst into tears of relief. I also felt intense happiness when I was told that this bundle of joy was a little girl. She had a huge mop of black hair and looked absolutely gorgeous. Nick took the train to London the next morning and was delighted when he saw his daughter and first child. We agreed that her first name would be Azuka – it means 'family support is more valued than money'. This was his Igbo name, one that can be given to both girls and boys. Her second name was Elizabeth.

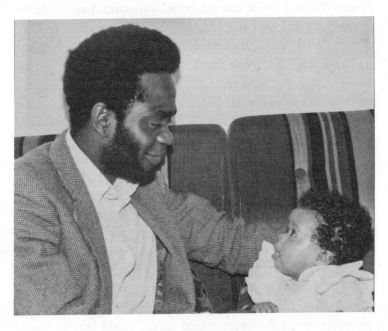

Nick and Azuka.

In January 1982, Regi wrote thanking me for the photo I sent, saying, 'Azuka looks a bit like your daddy and very hairy for a baby.' Pleased that she noted the resemblance, the other comment seemed a bit harsh. Not as shocking, though, as the Black woman who visited me in hospital, peered at the baby and said, 'She's really pretty, but what a shame about her flat nose. Just put a nose peg on it or pinch it every day to straighten it out.'

Sadly, after the birth, Nick admitted to me that he was married. Even though he was planning to get a divorce, I was angry and horrified and could no longer trust him. It was a dreadful period and one I couldn't discuss with my mother, probably because she had been through a much more difficult time. Whatever the reason, it was impossible to open up to her over the phone. I could talk to friends face to face, but I didn't want to distress her with the situation.

(Nick and I were to remain on reasonably friendly terms for over twelve years. He occasionally saw Azuka in England prior to his departure for Nigeria in 1983, where he resumed academic activities at his university and ultimately became a professor. I would visit Nigeria with Azuka every year or two up until her teens, when we would stay with him and his second wife, who I got on very well with. Later, there was a half-brother and half-sister, but as Azuka got older, the relationship with her father became less close. In 2014, Azuka's sister informed her of his death in Nigeria while he was staying at a hotel on academic business. Azuka and I were both thirty-three years old when our fathers died.)

My friend Sue had been correct in wondering how I would manage with less sleep. As it happened, there was one occasion when I missed a feed in the night due to sheer exhaustion. My painful, swollen breasts woke me with a start, and I dashed into Azuka's room. There, I saw a sleeping baby sucking away at nothing – the guilt was horrendous. So, I sat next to the cot and the minute I saw a movement I immediately picked her up and put her onto my breast. She literally lunged at it, not taking a break for ages. I never realised a baby could go so long without a proper breath.

Life with a small child could at times be much tougher than I had expected, but Azuka was very placid and sweet. The support of friends and my previous health visiting experience all helped enormously. Even though I had continued working until just a few days before her delivery, there was still pressure on me to return as early as possible as a sickle cell nurse counsellor, now that we'd got a screening programme up and running. Against my deepest wishes, I reluctantly went back to work when Azuka was only nine weeks of age and it upset me for a long time. It was Dolores who came to my rescue, as she became Azuka's childminder for the first two years of her life. She also acted as a mother figure to me and provided much-needed guidance, support, humour and friendship.

I remember in those early days, wrapping up this tiny baby to take to Dolores's home and trying to warm the car up in the freezing cold first thing in the morning; I didn't want to be bringing a nine-week-old out into this vicious weather. I'd sit in the car with her in the backseat, waiting for the wretched car to heat up and feeling so angry. One thing that consoled me was giving her a morning and evening breastfeed until she was six months old. Being a single parent, thank God for my friends around me.

I wished my mum could have visited and given me much-needed support, but for whatever reason that never happened, as she only stayed once for a few days at the time of Azuka's christening. This was the only occasion that Azuka, Nick, Mum and I were to be gathered together. My sister Marion remembers a similar experience. Although they lived in the same town, Mum never came to see Marion at the hospital following the birth of her first child. We can never know what psychological issues were causing her to react in this way to the birth of her grandchildren.

On a positive note, when I was pregnant, I'd had my own screening at Queen Charlotte's Hospital. Here, the consultant haematologist, Dr Elizabeth Letsky, was ahead of many of her peers in establishing routine sickle cell and thalassaemia screening and genetic counselling in pregnancy. Having been so recently pregnant, once back at work it did make it easier for me to empathise with the fears of parents-to-be.

The first separation Azuka and I experienced was when she was two and I attended a one-week sickle cell conference in Toronto, Canada. During this period, she lived with Dolores and her family while I stayed with friends and their young family in Toronto. They totally understood how much I missed her and my feelings of guilt. I will never forget their kindness when they insisted that I use their phone, without charge, to make daily international calls to chat to her. It was always wonderful to hear Azuka's high-pitched chatter. On my return, she came running towards me so fast that our heads nearly collided as I knelt to give her a kiss and a hug.

Life became easier for the next few years, thanks to her attending an excellent local nursery. Similar to many other working parents, I had quite a shock when she left the nursery to start full-time education, and I struggled to find appropriate childcare after school and during the holidays.

Our visits to Nigeria started when Azuka was about three and a half years of age. I was determined that she would visit the country, her father and the Anionwu family from as early in childhood as possible. She said:

> I always think of Nigeria like the *Wizard of Oz*, when Dorothy is in Kansas and it's black and white and cold and stoic. Then it goes to Oz and it's colourful and warm. That's what Nigeria reminds me of. So, the Irish white side of your family is a bit like Kansas, black and white and a bit cold. Having said that, I always got on well with my cousins in Wolverhampton, but I needed to be there for a bit before feeling relaxed enough to chat and play with them. Then going to Nigeria, and it's just a burst of colour and energy and friendliness and love and feelings. I think Nigerians and Africans as a whole have a good way of making people feel at home and part of their family. That always struck me instantly. I felt a sense of belonging, which I'm sure you felt when you first went there.

Azuka loved Nigerian food, such as the large snails, okra soup and meat stews. She copied others in chewing down to the very last bit of the bone. As well as spending time with her father in Port Harcourt, we also travelled to Onitsha, where the Anionwu family made a tremendous fuss over her. One day we went to a traditional ceremony at Onitsha, and Azuka quickly appreciated the importance of sitting quietly during the libations. She was particularly fascinated with the sight of the coral bead necklaces and bracelets worn by so many people. At one point, she nudged me and pointed to a titled elder woman sitting next to her, and I saw that she had 'Azuka' tattooed on her arm. It was the first time my daughter had seen someone with the same name as herself. At this same event, someone observed Azuka taking a few sips of palm wine from a nearby cup and becoming slightly tipsy. She couldn't understand why I made her drink lots of water.

We also stayed with my cousin Joy and her family in Lagos, where Azuka had a wonderful time with her little cousins. I was quite the anxious mother, as this was her first trip abroad. Joy quickly sorted me out by telling me to get some well-earned rest during my stay. She also told me to get used to the fact that, from now on, Azuka would be busy playing with her cousins. It was just the right type of parenting lesson that I needed.

At the end of our wonderful trip, she cried her little heart out on the day of our departure for England. Not quite four, she plaintively asked me who she was going to play with back home. In fact, she also loved our visits to friends in the UK, who were a great source of company for her and support for me. These included Janet, Ann and Steve, Ursula, Sue, as well as Alan and his wife, Kay. They all regularly welcomed us into their homes, and Azuka grew up enjoying being able to play with their children.

When I was actively involved with sickle cell issues, I was also determined that Azuka would come with me to as many events as possible, both at home and abroad. 'With your sickle cell stuff, I went around with you a lot. When I was younger, I could see you as a campaigner and I remember once when I wished I had sickle cell. Also, I remember playing with the dolls in the nursery and a vivid memory is of me giving one particular doll a blood transfusion,' she said. We travelled far afield to countries such as Jamaica, Bermuda, the French Caribbean isles of Guadeloupe and Martinique, Nigeria and Holland. My ability to speak French resulted in requests to run sickle courses in Martinique and Guadeloupe.

In 1990, a comprehensive sickle cell centre was opened in Guadeloupe's capital of Pointe-à-Pitre. There was intense local pride that it was the first such French centre, and ahead of 'la Métropole' – that is, the European territory of France. When we visited, Azuka attended a local school where none of the children spoke English, although some of the teachers did. She was the centre of attention and still remembers the friends she made, regardless of language barriers. Her other abiding memory was of the tasty and nutritious food that she ate at the school, including guavas. My memories were of the amazing hospitality, discussions, sea-bathing and dancing to Zouk and Biguine music.

We would also take regular drives to Wolverhampton so Azuka could see her grandmother and the family – for which Azuka is grateful:

> You always made an effort to keep in touch with her so that I would know her and that side of the family. You loved her and were very devoted to her and worked hard to keep in contact with her. Neither of you were that tactile, unlike how you've been with me. She was quiet and always surrounded by a lot of books. As I was also shy, we never seemed to be able speak to each other at great length. She loved animals and sometimes I sensed she liked them more than people.

Azuka's observations on Ken were interesting:

> He was always very tactile, playful and friendly towards me. But as I got older, I sensed there were some bad vibes and a history there between you two. I remember one occasion, it was either Christmas or Easter, and he got a bit drunk and started talking about the past. I could

sense your body change and you got very tense, which is something that I'd rarely seen you do. The expression on your face changed and we left soon after.

Ken definitely went out of his way to be charming to both Azuka and myself during these day trips to Wolverhampton. Prior to my departure for London, he would check the oil and water and repeatedly go over the directions to the motorway. My sister Marion recalled that as a teenager, even she knew the route off by heart.

Azuka did remember, however:

As a kid I liked to suck my thumb and stroke my eyebrow. You have lovely eyebrows that I always wanted to stroke, but when I stroked your left eyebrow, you'd wince in pain. When I was a bit older, you explained that Ken used to beat you and had once hit you so hard that you fell into the fireplace and cut your eyebrow. It is a pain that has never really gone away. If you touch there it hurts. But also, I wonder if it's an emotional scar, as well.

Chapter 36:
A Tough Role

It soon became clear that my role at the screening centre as counsellor would embrace everything from cradle to grave. In the early 1980s, up to three of our local patients died each year, and there would be other losses among those I knew through the Sickle Cell Society. Dr Ade Olujohungbe was a consultant haematologist and medical advisor for the organisation (he had the illness and sadly died in 2013, weeks before his long-awaited fiftieth birthday). He was so friendly, intelligent and extremely committed to improving the quality of treatment for the condition; his passing shocked so many people.

This was the worst aspect of my work, and I would dread the call that somebody had died or was dangerously ill. They were always so young, and the shock and grief of their family and friends was utterly heartbreaking. One would be dear Francis, who died in his early forties and had only just started to come to terms with his illness. I would often visit bereaved families, and I remember one such visit was to a Nigerian diplomat whose very young daughter had recently died. He suddenly started to weep, saying that fathers missed their children as much as their mothers; it was heart-rending.

Sometimes Misha asked me to act as an intermediary for doctors finding it difficult to cope with different cultural expressions of grief. This could range from huge numbers of family and friends angrily demanding answers, to people howling in utter anguish. One doctor opened up to me about his dread of dealing with these multiple displays of grief, as he had never come across it before he came to London. His own words were: 'My middle-class white background and my medical training haven't prepared me for such powerful expressions of loss.'

After a few joint meetings with bereaved relatives, we took some time to discuss his observations. His main reflections centred on how I listened with respect and didn't interrupt, regardless of occasional accusations against the hospital of racism and/or negligent care. In fact, I would make sure that the family knew where to make a complaint. Questions were answered immediately and where not all of the information was available, a promise was made to investigate further. He noticed how at ease I seemed to be with various cultural attitudes towards death and dying. Of interest to me was the way he pointed out how members of the group would often determine when it was time to stop talking and/or challenge those who they thought were being too brusque with me.

I said that it was important not to feel personally challenged. Time was required to ensure that possibly years of pent-up emotions could be expressed at this time of utter shock and grief. It was often young Black individuals who had died suddenly. Our in-depth discussions allowed us both to avoid tiptoeing around certain issues. He revealed that he had never really understood why so many Black relatives and friends came to the hospital, nor why some acted so aggressively. I asked him to consider whether he was actually scared of Black people when they acted in such a raw, emotional and challenging manner, to which he admitted he was.

It was an uphill struggle to convince a range of local and national authorities about the significance of the condition. So, imagine my surprise when in 1985 a letter arrived asking if I would accept an MBE in the forthcoming New Year's Honours list. After some consideration, I wrote back thanking the powers that be for the recognition but refusing it on the grounds that government support was needed to improve sickle cell services throughout the country.

There would eventually be some secretarial support in Brent, but it had taken until 1985 to secure extra funding for the appointment of two health visitors, Marvelle and Nina, to assist with the increased sickle cell work. Nina, who spoke Gujarati, also helped to develop awareness of thalassaemia within the local South Asian community.

All this activity generated even greater interest from the media. In June 1984, the Channel 4 television programme *Black on Black*, produced by Trevor Phillips, featured weekly items over a three-week period. Celebrities were also filmed donating blood. A direct result of this was a phone call from someone introducing himself as Garth Crooks, a football player for Tottenham Hotspur and England. He had been disappointed that an overseas match had made it impossible for him to take part in the TV programme, but he now wanted to organise an annual gala dinner and dance so that he and his famous friends could help raise funds for sickle cell awareness. Garth invited me to become a member of his planning committee, which was meeting the following week. I enquired where and Garth replied, 'White Hart Lane.' I asked, 'What number?' After a short silence, he burst out laughing, saying it was clear that I didn't follow the game.

If there had ever been doubts about the need for a specialist service of this kind, the amazing response we had speaks for itself. By 1987, more than 3,000 people had attended screening and genetic counselling sessions, with over 50 per cent being self-referrals. In 1979, I was in contact with seventy individuals with sickle cell disease and by 1988 this had risen to 382. Of these, 112 were under the age of sixteen years.[1]

My MPhil degree had now been converted to a PhD and, by late 1986, I had completed the research for my thesis. My problem was affording a computer at home to type it all up, so I went into work to do it at the weekends. I would drive Azuka to stay overnight with my friend Ursula, where she loved being in the company of her children. Even so, I was wracked with guilt at these frequent short separations and promised her that when it was all finished, we would make a trip to Disneyland in Los Angeles. So it was that having at last been awarded my PhD, we spent Christmas of 1988 in America. Here, I was able to watch my seven-year-old daughter have one of the best holidays of her life.

Chapter 37:

Moving On

All seemed to be going swimmingly in Brent until an unexpected and unwelcome sea change occurred around 1987. Misha appointed a new consultant, which resulted in two significant developments. The first was welcome, as by 1988 it was the result of an expansion of newborn screening throughout the North West Thames Region. The funding obtained by North West Thames Regional Health Authority enabled the appointment of more health visiting and administrative staff. The second, and much less pleasant, was the change in culture due to a different management style. In contrast to Misha's inclusive style, I gradually sensed one of harassment, bullying, criticism and control. There was now a hierarchical atmosphere, with micromanagement, memos galore and checks on everything. I can laugh now, but sometimes it felt as though I needed permission even to go to the toilet. Weirdly, this took me back to how my stepfather had made me feel, a dark place indeed, as I felt like I couldn't do anything right.

What particularly saddened and confused me was how my relationship with Misha suffered, as she appeared to step back from it all (our relationship would only recover after my departure). At around the same time I went to Nigeria to co-run Professor Akinyanju's Lagos-based annual sickle course. At one point he took me aside and urged me to take six months off work, as this would be essential if I was ever to complete my PhD thesis. My subsequent request for paid study leave was turned down flat, which made me extremely angry. I decided to take the six months off with three months' paid sick leave to have an overdue hysterectomy for fibroids, followed by three months' unpaid leave. I just about survived financially due to the King's Fund coming to my rescue again, with a £1000 grant and by signing on for benefits.

Coming round from surgery, I saw the wonderful Professor Luzzatto was peering down at me and asking how I felt. He was in charge of the haematology department at Hammersmith Hospital, and I suddenly felt very safe. The next day a friend brought seven-year-old Azuka to visit me and I could see my daughter's anxious glance at the intravenous drip in my arm. Worsening tensions, which also affected Nina, marred my return to work and I don't think the award of a PhD improved the atmosphere that much. It was probably one of the most stressful periods of my working life, and Nina recalls us both crying once in the human resources department.

We decided to seek advice and support from our union, which led to us taking out a grievance. This shook a member of the HR staff, who said they had never had to deal with one taken out against anyone so senior. Well, I thought bitterly, this is a chance for you to gain some experience. The management tried frantically to resolve the issues by suggesting alternative management structures and work locations. They genuinely seemed to value our lengthy involvement in developing highly acclaimed services.

In the midst of all of this, I began experiencing severe headaches and took myself off to the occupational health service. I was diagnosed with high blood pressure, so I immediately made a decision to leave the job and as early as possible, even before I had obtained another post. Azuka was still young, and my family history of strokes was such that I determined no job was worth the risk. At least I had my health visiting qualification, and I would be very happy to return to that career.

There was, of course, tremendous sadness at the thought of leaving the world of sickle cell and all of the families I knew so well. It was made even more difficult when a group of them asked me to reconsider my decision. A friend commented: 'I think for you it was a good move, but it was a big loss for the Brent Centre.' Ursula, a friend and a mother of a daughter with sickle cell anaemia, reflected: 'It kind of saddened me that that was the case, because who else was better placed to represent us, parents of children with sickle cell, the Black community, the cause that you were fighting for?'

Chapter 38:

Forging Ahead

Having made up my mind to leave and look for a post as a health visitor, I received a phone call that was to change everything and totally lift my spirits. It was from Professor Marcus Pembrey, Consultant Clinical Geneticist at the University of London's Institute of Child Health and Great Ormond Street Hospital for Children. He wanted to apologise about being away on the day I was due to come and talk to his MSc in clinical genetics students.

There must have been something in the way I spoke that alerted him to my dejected state of mind. It didn't take him long to discover my plans to quit and, to my eternal joy, he asked if I would consider working at the institute. Marcus was aware of my ambition to establish a course on multi-ethnic aspects of screening and genetic counselling. As he later reflected, 'The lesson from that quite simply is you never know when you're having a conversation what effect it might have, you just do what you think is the right thing to do.'

He explained:

Haemoglobinopathies screening was an important part of genetic services and a significant issue that we weren't covering at the institute. When I arrived here, we were isolated from the community. A sort of ivory tower, both clinically and in research, and it was important to try and break that down. It happened that I carried beta thalassaemia, even though I apparently don't come from the right ethnic group. So, this showed I was beginning to think that things are not always the way they seem. You can't pigeonhole people. Having beta thalassaemia in the family encouraged me to study the subject when I was a student and that got me into haemoglobinopathies research.

Then I was out in Saudi Arabia showing that they didn't suffer as badly from sickle cell disease, due to their raised fetal haemoglobin. I wanted to go on and do something similar here, but nobody seemed to be doing it. You raised the ethnicity issues. There was a part of me that felt, why should haemoglobinopathies be nothing to do with clinical genetics? So, I think you were helping me with a political agenda. It didn't take me long to realise that we were thinking alike. So, you were a breath of fresh air and a dream come true.

In the autumn of 1990, I attended a formal selection interview in front of an impressive panel of academics at the UCL Great Ormond Street Institute of Child Health and was appointed Lecturer in Community Genetic Counselling. The next seven years at the Institute of Child Health would prove to be incredibly happy and productive ones, although I vividly recall sitting alone at a desk on my first day. Looking at the blank pad of paper, I wondered to myself, *what on earth have you got yourself into?* Then I picked up the phone to book various speakers, received enthusiastic responses and immediately felt better.

Marcus's management style also suited me down to the ground. As he commented, it was characterised by putting all of his effort into attracting the right people and then 'not really managing anybody'. When I hesitantly mentioned an invitation I had recently received to visit Guadeloupe for two weeks in October 1990, Marcus was actually pleased to hear that not only would I be a guest of honour at the opening of the Sickle Cell Centre, but also that I would jointly run a course. The second example of Marcus's refreshing management style was when I asked for an annual leave card to book time off for Azuka's half-term holiday and discovered their non-existence in the department. 'One of the first things I did was to abolish holiday forms because the senior staff didn't have to fill them in. It seemed wrong, and it actually achieved nothing because my main problem was getting people to take their holidays.' Both illustrated a seismic and heartening shift away from the work culture that I had recently left.

There was also a keen respect for nurses, and one nurse's influence soon became apparent. During a meeting, we were talking about some aspect of the profession and Marcus kept referring to somebody called Sue. It took some time for the penny to drop. When I asked if he was talking about the iconic Sue Pembrey, he said, 'Yes, you do realise that she is my sister?' Sue had become well-known in nursing due to her research on the role of the ward sister. She had also set up and run the famous Oxford Nursing Development Unit at the Radcliffe Infirmary.

My first contact with her had been as far back as July 1971, when she spoke at a conference on private practice organised by the Young Socialist Medical Association and reported in *Needle* magazine. Sue had spoken on agency nursing, and argued that the attraction for nurses was more the flexible hours rather than the money and that that should be a lesson for the NHS.

I titled my two-week course 'Genetic Counselling for the Community – A Multi-Ethnic Approach'. It would focus on the similarities and differences faced by couples at risk of genetic disorders such as sickle cell disease, thalassaemia, cystic fibrosis and Tay-Sachs disease. The latter progressively destroys nerve cells in the brain and spinal cord, resulting in death at about the age of five. There is a significantly higher incidence of the illness in people of Eastern European Ashkenazi Jewish descent, although it is also found in other populations.

This is exactly what had always fascinated me about these inherited conditions: it's generally well recognised that all have a higher incidence in certain ethnic groups. Those at increased risk of the various thalassaemia syndromes include populations originating from the Mediterranean, the Middle and Far East, as well as South Asia. Cystic fibrosis is most commonly found in people of white Northern European origin.[1]

Many health professionals thought that only certain groups were at risk of a particular genetic disorder. The classic misunderstanding is that cystic fibrosis was only seen in white people, thalassaemia in Greek and Turkish-Cypriots, Tay-Sachs in Ashkenazi Jews and sickle cell in the Black community. Less well known was that all of these conditions are also seen in other groups, although usually to a lesser extent. Between them, all these genetic disorders impact on most communities in this country.

I ran twenty courses between 1991 and 1997. A total of 296 people attended, who were mainly midwives, haemoglobinopathy counsellors and genetic nurses. There were also doctors, family planning nurses and health visitors. Most came from the UK, with the majority from the North Thames Region of London, and there was at least one overseas participant on each course. On day one, each participant would be given a thick dossier of information on everything we'd be covering. Nowadays, I would just be able to give them a list of website links, but back then I had a fantastic secretary who would make sure the dossier was still relevant, so if new screening programmes came along, we'd add in the information. Even years later, people would say they'd still dig into it for facts.

I quickly became aware of the many sensitive issues that could affect my students due to their own experiences or belief systems. These included the ethics surrounding perceptions of disability and the option of prenatal diagnosis and termination for an affected unborn baby. During the first course, I realised that midwives were constantly comparing their varied experiences with the recently introduced Bart's test. I had never heard of it, so asked them to explain further and, oh boy, they did just that. It turned out to be a new way of identifying pregnant women with a possible increased risk of having a baby with Down's syndrome.

Many thought it had been introduced too quickly and felt unprepared for their role in informing the women about the exact details of this test compared to other forms of screening. As a result, they were very anxious and strongly urged me to include a session about it in future courses. The whole topic of screening for the condition was taken on board and I started including a speaker from the Down's Syndrome Association in the programme.

Another speaker was Dr Elizabeth Dormandy, who explained:

My responsibility was education and training across thirty-odd hospitals in North Thames. I could see that you were aiming to equip people to offer support, help and counselling to women and their families from a broad range of backgrounds and perspectives. I found that incredibly exciting. I had previously worked in the laboratories where everything was clear-cut, yes or no. Your course enabled people to think about screening from the perspective of people being offered it. We knew the uptake of Down's syndrome screening varied hugely from 30 per cent in some areas to 90 per cent in other areas. This variation occurred year on year, and it was obvious there was something going on other than women's decisions.

I realised how important it was that you got parents and people with the condition to come and talk to course participants. As a white liberal, I was sort of aware of different people's perspectives on ethnicity, but also a bit scared of it. I was able to see the similarities and appreciate the differences, and it gave me confidence to talk about it. I learned that we all come with different prejudices – some we are aware of and some we are not, but we need to work through it.

One of the most vivid examples that came to light on the course was an account from a midwife. One morning, she had collected a large quantity of patients' notes in preparation for a busy antenatal clinic. Seeing that the first patient had an Indian name, she put it lower down the pile to avoid having to immediately address 'language and cultural problems'.

When the woman's turn eventually came, the midwife was mortified to discover that she was an Oxford graduate and medically qualified.

This incident shocked the midwife, exposing as it did her own stereotypical and negative assumptions. It spurred her on to realise that she needed to seek the advice, resources and challenges the course could offer. There began to be a waiting list for the courses, as well as many requests to speak about them – more than I could fulfil – from far and wide.

In order to disseminate the philosophy of the course more widely, I obtained a grant from the Department of Health to produce a 23-minute video and leaflet. The video, which was produced in 1993, was called *From Chance to Choice* and was described as 'a multi-ethnic approach to community genetics: the role of the primary health care team.'

I also became a member of the Gene Therapy Advisory Committee (GTAC) in 1993 and the newly formed Human Genetics Commission (HGC) in 1999. The latter was steered by two incredibly eminent and charismatic Scots – the Glaswegian Baroness Helena Kennedy, QC (who was the chair) and her deputy, Alexander McCall Smith, Professor of Medical Law at the University of Edinburgh. He was also a bestselling author of works that included The No. 1 Ladies' Detective Agency series, set in Botswana. Other committees that I belonged to during this period included the Department of Health's Antenatal Subgroup of the National Screening Group and the Nuffield Council on Bioethics Working Party on Genetic Screening.

While at the institute, it was also good to continue with my sickle cell interests in many different ways. I was able to resume genetic counselling by providing local support to colleagues in Islington and Camden. These sessions took place at the Sickle Cell and Thalassaemia Centre, the paediatric and antenatal clinics at the Whittington Hospital and the prenatal diagnosis unit at University College Hospital, London.

In 1991, I was invited to become a member of the Department of Health's Standing Medical Advisory Committee (SMAC) working party on sickle cell, thalassaemia and other haemoglobinopathies. The report was published in 1993 and contained sixty-two recommendations, but the only one that received funding was the production of a national haemoglobinopathy result card. However, the publication did raise the profile of the issues of concern to patients, families and professionals.

The BBC Radio 4 *Today* programme contacted me at an unearthly hour one morning with a request to come into the studio to comment on some development in genetics and sickle cell disease. I said that unfortunately it would be impossible because of childcare issues. There was a slightly surprised response of, 'Oh, really?', followed by an offer to interview me over the phone at work. I agreed and, sometime after it was over, I told Marcus the story. He burst out laughing saying: 'Elizabeth, you don't seem to realise, there would be people here who'd kill to get to the studio to be on that programme.'

The world of collaborating in research projects opened up for me in a way that I hadn't really envisaged. My room at the institute was at the end of a corridor, and the walk to the kitchen for a coffee enabled me to bump into staff from so many disciplines. This included public health, statistics, epidemiology and genetics. Suitable calls for research bids would be mentioned and meetings arranged to consider putting in a joint application. The discussions were intellectually stimulating and provided an opportunity to input ideas drawn from my NHS nursing and community sickle cell and thalassaemia experience. Such collaboration was also immensely enjoyable and gave me increased confidence to develop research and publication skills. This turned out to be an extremely productive period for me, as I was a member of several research teams. Bids for various projects were awarded a total of nearly £1 million from the NHS and the Department of Health. When I was promoted in 1994, Marcus pointed out: 'Well, it's not easy to get a promotion to a senior lecturer here.' Those seven happy and fulfilling years at the institute were to transform me and restore my self-confidence – so much so that my thoughts turned to advancing my career in a way that would help our family of two.

Azuka was now a teenager and, as for many parents, it was incomprehensible and painful for me to witness a seeming overnight change in the relationship with my previously loving and sweet child. It certainly wasn't helped by our equally obstinate personalities. Azuka felt very lonely coming home after school to an empty flat. I constantly encouraged her to attend some of the varied extracurricular activities available to her but without success.

So we had the typical shouting, door-slamming and ulti-matums, and I wouldn't wish the experience on anybody. After one row, Azuka started blasting out the sounds of Tupac, the late US rapper. This particular song, 'Hit 'Em Up', is probably one of the best-known 'diss' songs. There was a bitter ongoing East Coast/West Coast rivalry, and the lyrics were targeted at his enemies, Notorious B.I.G. (aka Biggie) and Junior M.A.F.I.A. Suffice it to say, it was done to provoke a reaction from me, as it is riddled with profane language. It worked. I snapped and threatened to remove all of her Tupac tapes if she didn't turn it off immediately. That also worked.

There was nobody either of us could immediately turn to when tensions arose. Once again, it never crossed my mind to pick up the phone and speak to my mother. And there were no relatives living close enough to us who could provide an immediate refuge for Azuka when she felt lonely and overwhelmed, or when a crisis loomed. Fortunately, on one such occasion it was half-term, so Azuka could travel to stay with my sister and her children in Wolverhampton – thank you, Marion – and it provided the breathing space the pair of us so badly needed.

I didn't grow up with the opportunity to pick up hints about parenting in close quarters. Friends like Ursula realised that this might be part of the problem:

> What was great was the way you would explain things to Azuka. I didn't think you were too strict; you hardly ever lost your temper with her and you seemed to prefer giving an explanation. But I came from a family with so many of us and I think you were sometimes wary of setting stricter boundaries. I don't think it was anything major; it was just that I think you only had one child and hadn't got that experience of dealing with challenges and temper tantrums. I'd think, God almighty, child, just leave me alone kind of thing! You know, there were times when I would have just taken charge of Azuka and dealt with her, but I didn't want to interfere. So, I think not having had that experience and being on your own, it came out sometimes in your parenting.

During Azuka's turbulent teenage years while I was working at the Institute of Child Health, I discovered that a colleague was going through a similar experience. We formed a mutual self-help group and found it very cathartic to discuss our latest adolescent outbursts and run-ins. Drama and musical theatre were to provide a sanctuary for Azuka, and a wonderful English teacher recognised her abilities and acted as her mentor, fortunately.

However, in order to improve our relationship, I realised the need to spend more time with her and looked to secure a more local position. In the autumn of 1997, I was appointed as Dean of the School of Adult Nursing at Thames Valley University (TVU), now the University of West London. For two years I would manage fifty-three nurse tutors and immerse myself in the world of nursing and higher education. It would prove to be quite a culture shock, but ultimately I settled happily into a post that brought me back to my preferred calling.

After six months, I was awarded a Chair in Nursing. The positive impact of this appointment on others was quite an eye-opener, as some of my colleagues remember. Ramesh, a senior nurse lecturer, said:

> You were the first Black person to be in such a high position here and were very genuine. You came in with ideas and encouraged us enormously to stretch ourselves clinically and academically, and that was what people wanted. I wanted to publish and sought your advice, and you immediately said, 'Yes, come and see me.' For the first time I felt supported, and after just two sessions with you I managed to complete the paper, which was published in 1998.

Felicia, a director of nursing, explained: 'One big wow factor for me was that you're a professor, a Black professor of nursing!' While Baba, a consultant haematologist and now a professor, said:

> It helped a lot of people, be they doctors, nurses or others, who saw you as a role model, even though they had never met you. I and other people felt very proud that you had progressed to the level of a professor and a major nursing role, as well as making such an impact on sickle cell in the UK. You actually wanted to be associated with this person and I loved the name, which was a Nigerian name, Anionwu! It gave me hope that we can make it, as well.

Although up to my eyes with management matters, I was determined to continue with my sickle cell interests. These included teaching, research and community activities, as well as the securing of a fortnightly clinical attachment to a haematology ward in a west London hospital. I declined the offer of a sister's uniform from the director of nursing, instead requesting from him one for a staff nurse. He told me later that he couldn't quite get over the shock of seeing a professor of nursing working on a ward. It was a great experience and also set an example to students and the few nurse tutors who had been reluctant to have their own clinical link.

Retaining my involvement with community and policy aspects of sickle cell was of particular importance. This was achieved through collaborating with Karl Atkin, Professor of Sociology at the University of York. We also shared a keen interest in the historical milestones that had led to sickle cell and thalassaemia gradually coming in from the cold and onto the NHS agenda. The best example was the inclusion of universal newborn and antenatal screening in the government's NHS Plan in 2000.[2]

Within a few years all babies in England, regardless of ethnic origin, were being screened for sickle cell disease – an incredible feat achieved through the dynamic leadership of Archbishop John Sentamu, who chaired the advisory committee, and Dr Allison Streetly, director of the programme. We wrote about these developments in a book called *The Politics of Sickle Cell and Thalassaemia*, published by Open University Press in 2001.

Karl also pointed out that at dissemination meetings with doctors and policy-makers, the top table would be predominantly white while the audience was predominantly Black – and that even in the sickle cell world, some people had difficulty with the idea of an articulate and educated Black woman:

> You were always such a good chair at those community meetings. This was a highly politicised world where you really had to have credibility with that audience. You broke that mould and I think that was incredibly important . . . [but] from seeing you in the many meetings over the years I could see that it was a struggle . . . People looking to undermine you, and that's wearing over years and years. But in some ways, you could use that to your advantage as well, because you gave credibility to the communities. It also meant you were slightly on the outside, which is not a bad thing.

Chapter 39:

The Inspiring Mrs Mary Seacole

Soon after I started work as Dean of the School of Adult Nursing at TVU, I made a point of talking to groups of student nurses, as it was crucial to hear directly from them about how the course was going and to obtain feedback about their clinical placement experiences. One student talked about being unfairly treated and wanted advice on how to handle it. I mentioned how Mary Seacole, the Victorian Jamaican-Scottish nurse, had overcome rejection when her offer to go and care for British soldiers in the Crimean War had been turned down. A sea of blank faces looked back at me, and it was obvious that not one of the twenty students had heard of her.

I systematically quizzed all future groups only to find that, apart from a handful of students, there was a widespread lack of knowledge (Ramesh, a senior nurse lecturer, said: 'I had never heard of Mary Seacole until you came on board. You not only raised my awareness, but also that of the whole nursing faculty.' Elaine, a retired head of a nursing school, commented: 'I had never heard of Mary Seacole throughout my entire nursing career. I taught student nurses and since I had never heard of her, the entire school never heard of her.')

It made me wonder why we weren't taught about her, and I felt my anger rise because here's an example of the mixed-race woman written out of history; she was well-known in Victorian media, so there's no excuse for her having been forgotten. In the nineteenth century, British officers would often marry women from the countries where they were stationed, but at some point attitudes shifted and a racist sense of absolute superiority over Black and brown-skinned people pervaded.

Mary Jane Grant Seacole had a particular resonance for me. Proud of her Jamaican and Scottish heritage, she condemned slavery and refused to accept discrimination while creating compassionate and skilful nursing care. Because she'd never been mentioned once throughout all of my years of training and nursing, I only learned about Mary in 1984, at the launch of a new edition of her 1857 autobiography, *Wonderful Adventures of Mrs Seacole in Many Lands*.

Mary's mother was one of many women who were notable doctresses and whose expertise was recognised throughout Jamaica, and from her Mary learned 'a great deal of Creole medical art'. In 1836, Mary wed an Englishman, Edwin Horatio Hamilton Seacole, but their marriage was to last only eight years. Her husband was delicate, and Mary nursed him until his death in 1844. (Oral history recounted through the ages by the Seacole family suggests that he might have been the son of Admiral Nelson and Emma, Lady Hamilton.)

Mary suffered another loss with the death of her mother, but struggled on as a widow by taking on diverse business ventures (with varying degrees of success) and 'gained a reputation as a skilled nurse and doctress, and [her] house was always full of invalid officers . . .' The bulk of Mary's autobiography reveals her feisty nature and determination to overcome whatever barriers she came across. She displayed powerful networking skills and wasn't afraid to seek help from those she knew at the highest echelons of medicine and the military. What I find particularly appealing is Mary's refusal to be viewed as an inferior person on the basis of her skin colour, telling an American: 'But I must say that I don't altogether appreciate your friend's kind wishes with respect to my complexion . . . and as to his offer of bleaching me, I should, even if it were practicable, decline it without any thanks.'

When Mary learned about the Crimean War and read about the shocking maladministration and appalling nursing care, she reacted to the call for nurses to work under Florence Nightingale at Scutari Barracks Hospital in Turkey. Arriving at Southampton, Mary missed Florence Nightingale by a few days, as she was already on her way to Scutari with a group of thirty-eight nurses. Seacole unsuccessfully sought sponsorship to travel to the Crimea and also applied to be part of the second group of nurses about to depart for Turkey, but was informed that sufficient numbers had been recruited. Mary thought that even if there had been a vacancy, she wouldn't have been the nurse chosen to fill it.

What continues to impress me immensely is the manner in which Mary responded to the rejections of her offers of help. It stands as a useful example to others who find themselves in that situation today. First, it illustrates the deep hurt that racism can cause an individual, wondering as she wept, 'Was it possible that American prejudices against colour had some root here?' Secondly, it provides a case study of how one determined 49-year-old Victorian woman of colour overcame despair at the numerous attempts to thwart her ambitions. By 1855, Mary had raised sufficient funds to travel to the Crimea, establishing the 'British Hotel' very close to the war zone with a store and canteen. Mary also ran a morning dispensary before visiting sick and wounded soldiers in their huts or on the battlefield.

After the war ended suddenly in 1856, Mary returned to London, where she was declared bankrupt. Key figures in the military and the media, together with members of the Royal Family, rallied round to ensure she wasn't destitute. One stunning example was the four-day Seacole Fund Grand Military Festival held in July 1857. A total of 80,000 people attended the gala, and it was widely reported in the Victorian media. Mary Seacole died aged seventy-six in London on 14 May 1881 as a result of 'apoplexy' or a stroke. Nearly a century later, she was virtually lost to history, to the extent that it wasn't even known whether she was buried in London or Jamaica.[1]

There is a wonderful article written in 1975 by Miss J. Elise Gordon, former editor of the *Nursing Mirror*, which reveals how she eventually solved this mystery.[2] In the early 1970s, she purchased a first edition of Mrs Seacole's autobiography in a London bookshop. Inside was a slip of paper with details that enabled Gordon to locate Mary's burial place in St Mary's Catholic Cemetery in Kensal Green, north-west London. The derelict grave was restored with a new headstone and reconsecrated on 20 November 1973, courtesy of many organisations. These included the British Commonwealth Nurses' War Memorial Fund, the Lignum Vitae Club (a London-based group of Jamaican women) and the UK Jamaican Nurses' Association.

In 1980, Ziggi Alexander and Audrey Dewjee undertook research for the Brent Library Services exhibition *Roots in Britain: Black and Asian Citizens from Elizabeth I to Elizabeth II*. The exhibition was launched at the end of October 1980 and included a panel about Mary Seacole. It was the demand for more information about Mary that led to Ziggi and Audrey being commissioned to produce a new edition of her autobiography in 1984. In his review, Clive Davis wrote: 'A cottage industry is beginning to develop around the exploits of "Mother Seacole", a Jamaican Creole who became a Victorian celebrity for her work as a nurse in the Crimean War and then sank into obscurity for the next hundred years or so.'[3] From the mid-1980s onwards, places and buildings began to be called after Mary Seacole in areas such as Reading, Leicester, Liverpool and London.

During my tenure as Dean, I hosted a series of lectures concerned with multi-ethnic aspects of nursing. Thinking of a name under which to host them, I deliberately chose Mary Seacole in order to raise awareness among those who had never heard of her. To launch the event, senior staff from the university kindly helped me to organise a multicultural concert at Ealing Town Hall held on 16 July 1998. It seemed to strike a chord, with the arrival of a huge crowd of over 400 people.

A year later there arose an unexpected opportunity to make the academic unit a full-time reality, as the management hierarchy of the College of Nursing was about to be restructured. My boss, Pro-Vice Chancellor Lois Crooke, stopped me one day by the stairs and said, 'Look, I know you're thinking of leaving.' This came as something of a surprise to me, although I realised that Lois was aware of how increasingly frustrated I was becoming due to horrendously time-consuming administrative responsibilities. She acknowledged that the opportunities I had been promised to undertake research had never materialised and assured me that she wanted me to stay on, requesting that I write my own job description.

So it was that on 1 September 1999, the Mary Seacole Centre for Nursing Practice was established at TVU. The objective of the centre was to 'enable the integration of a multi-ethnic philosophy into the process of nursing and midwifery recruitment, education, practice and research'. It appeared to me that there was a predominantly white Eurocentric focus in many of these areas (for example, the paucity of information in the curriculum about conditions such as sickle cell disease; an under-representation, in comparison to the local populations of Slough and Ealing, of students of African-Caribbean and South Asian origin and the near-absence of non-white images used in teaching. Tutors were aware of this, pointing out that they were virtually impossible to obtain from their local Medical Illustration Department).

We had been discussing how students are taught to recognise pallor, bruising and certain rashes in 'non-pink' skin. Many, many years ago I had read a newspaper account of a coroner's inquest into the death of a very young South Asian child in the north-east of England. It had followed a severe bleed after a tonsillectomy. The nurse had claimed to be unable to recognise increasing paleness, due to the brown colour of the child's skin. Other indicators of deterioration in health weren't identified, as the nurse had failed to undertake regular observations of the patient's pulse and respiration rates. Thankfully, there is now a higher profile on how this should be addressed in the curriculum.[4]

Over its eight-year lifetime, the centre was awarded more than a quarter of a million pounds for various research, recruitment and educational projects. There were three major pieces of work, including a campaign to attract nurses and midwives from diverse local ethnic groups (this was a successful community development project that began to redress the under-representation); multi-ethnic learning and teaching in nursing (an online educational resource developed for students and staff, which had an unexpected consequence – the demand for the inclusion of more information about Mary Seacole); and a study to monitor the impact of key diversity variables on the progression and transition into practice of student nurses. They included gender, country of birth, ethnicity and age. The research examined the outcome of 1,808 students enrolled on pre-registration nursing courses between 1999 and 2001. Findings of the study were published in 2008 in the *Journal of Advanced Nursing*.

Karl observed to me: 'I felt that you had always been perceived as a member of the Black community, rather than a well-qualified nurse, and a very successful one. It would have been around the late 1990s when the Establishment woke up and started to celebrate that.'

Chapter 40:

A Role Model

In 2001, I was awarded a CBE (Commander of the British Empire, or 'Cool, Black and Exceptional' as suggested by a friend) in The Queen's Birthday Honours List for my services to nursing. This award came as a great shock, and I still had reservations concerning the 'empire' bit. The empire doesn't exist anymore, and I don't understand why they can't change the names of the awards – there are enough people involved who could come up with a new word, and you have to ask, why haven't they done so? A significant number of would-be recipients have refused to accept the award because of that word.

It's like a slap in the face that Britain cannot acknowledge that this word 'empire' shouldn't be used. It's part of a history of one country ruling over another and, in the process, demeaning the subjects of that country. It's not just Britain – it was one country of many that colonised different parts of the world – and it seems obvious to humanity that you don't enslave others, and you don't drain other people's land of their gold and diamonds and other natural resources. Some people might say there were good aspects to the empire, but I say: it might have been good for you, my dear, but not so much for others. However, it was an important recognition for a Black nurse, in view of the difficulties that many faced in the profession.

Azuka and cousin-in-law Elaine came to the investiture at Buckingham Palace. My daughter wanted to know why Prince Charles had burst out laughing while he was pinning the medal on me. It had been due to the response I gave to his complimentary remarks about my colourful Nigerian gown: 'It has been said that I look pretty in pink!'

Then, in 2004 I flew to Belfast to receive a Fellowship of the Royal College of Nursing, a great accolade from my peers. This honour was for the development of nurse-led sickle cell and thalassaemia counselling services, and education and leadership in transcultural nursing.

In 2003, I was invited to join the Mary Seacole Memorial Statue Appeal. This had been founded by Lord Clive Soley after a group of Caribbean women in his west London constituency had asked him to accompany them to Mary Seacole's grave. There, they pointed out that this was her only memorial and wondered if he could help raise funds for a statue in her honour.

Around this time, general awareness about Mary began to improve for a variety of reasons. In 2002, the BBC launched a television poll to determine the 100 Greatest Britons; the overall winner was Sir Winston Churchill, yet not one single Black Briton featured on the list.[1] In response, in 2004, the commentator and activist Patrick Vernon organised an online vote called 100 Great Black Britons, and Mary Seacole was the winner; the subsequent publicity helped to raise her profile.[2] In an article in the *Guardian* on 14 February 2004, Nightingale biographer Mark Bostridge agreed that her selection was more than justified but acknowledged why so many of us are unhappy about Mary being referred to as the Black Nightingale: 'There is no doubt that in terms of practical nursing expertise, Seacole far outdistanced Nightingale's experience. Her work included preparing medicines, diagnosis and minor surgery.'

The next round of media attention came in 2005, with the bicentenary of Mary's year of birth. It kicked off with the announcement that historian Helen Rappaport had identified a lost portrait of Mary Seacole, which is now on display at the National Portrait Gallery in London. Then came the first major Seacole biography, written by Jane Robinson, a social historian specialising in the lives of women.[3] There was also the monograph *A Short History of Mary Seacole* that the Royal College of Nursing had commissioned me to write. It was designed to be a resource for nurses and students, and a copy was sent to the library of every college of nursing and midwifery in the UK.

In the summer of 2007, I made the decision to retire. About to turn sixty, I was now feeling the need to slow down a bit. After all, my working life had started at sixteen. I was also keen to have more control over my future activities. Moreover, Azuka – now working as a professional actress – had just given me the magnificent news that I would be a grandmother in the new year. To top it all, the university awarded me the title of Emeritus Professor in Nursing. So, there was a huge amount to celebrate, and my friends Nina and Majorie helped organise the most fantastic party to do just that.

In 2009, Martin Jennings was chosen as the artist to design the memorial statue for Mary Seacole. He is an internationally renowned sculptor whose body of work includes statues of poets Sir John Betjeman (at St Pancras International station) and Philip Larkin (in Hull). The site of the memorial statue is in the gardens of St Thomas' Hospital, London. Jennings explains that 'the sculpture represents her marching defiantly forward into an oncoming wind, as if confronting head-on some of the personal resistance she had constantly to battle . . .'

In that same year, the second only known photograph of Mary Seacole was rediscovered, together with a rare signature. It was found by Dr Geoffrey Day, then working as Fellows' and Eccles Librarian at Winchester College. The photo was in an elegant private Crimean War campaign scrapbook, compiled by former Coldstream Guards officer Ely Duodecimus Wigram (1802–1869). In 1916, it was presented to the Library of Winchester College by the then headmaster. The scrapbook contained incredible Crimean War memorabilia, including a collection of autographs and ten photographs of senior military personnel, plus one of Mary Seacole. Permission was given by Winchester College for the image to be used to raise funds for Mary's memorial statue.

In addition to twelve trustees and eleven patrons, the appeal selected over forty high-profile ambassadors from a wide variety of backgrounds. They included Dr Day, jazz musician Courtney Pine CBE, together with past Children's Laureates Malorie Blackman OBE and Michael Rosen. Also appointed were two Dutch Seacole researchers, Dr Corry Staring-Derks and Dr Jeroen Staring. Spending hours in the British Library, they unearthed a vast source of previously unknown Victorian newspaper coverage about Mary Seacole. *Nursing Standard* became the appeal's media partner and regularly included free one-page promotions about the charity.[4]

Planning consent was obtained from Lambeth Council in 2012, in spite of vociferous and continued opposition from a dozen or so people who were against it being installed at St Thomas' Hospital. They frequently cite it as an example of political correctness because they don't consider Seacole to be a nurse or even Black. It brings to mind Nobel

Prize-winning author Toni Morrison's comment to journalist Claudia Dreifus in 1994: 'What I think the political correctness debate is really about is the power to be able to define. The definers want the power to name. And the defined are now taking that power away from them.'

They are also concerned that, unlike Florence Nightingale, Mary Seacole didn't have any links to the hospital. The 2013 statement by Sir Hugh Taylor, Chairman of Guys and St Thomas' NHS Foundation Trust, is well worth a read: 'Mary Seacole was a pathfinder for the generations of people from Black and minority ethnic backgrounds who have served the NHS over the years and she remains a positive role model for the current generation. The Trust is proud to be hosting the statue, not least because it speaks to the diversity of our local population, our patients and the staff who work here.'

This view was admirably demonstrated countrywide in January 2013, when Michael Gove, then Education Secretary, threatened to exclude Mary Seacole (and others) from the proposed national curriculum. In the space of a few weeks, over 36,000 people had signed an online petition successfully demanding her inclusion. Organised by Operation Black Vote, the petition quickly went viral.

It seems to me that young children occasionally know more about Mary Seacole than some adults. A friend of mine informed me of the response of her six-year-old daughter to a query about what she had learned at school that day: 'We had a talk about two old dead nurses. One was Florence Nightingale and the other was Mary, umm, Mary Sequin.' When my granddaughter was seven, she informed me that she was being Mary Seacole as part of a class presentation on Victorians. Naturally I was absolutely delighted, although a bit taken aback when she asked if I had ever worked with her as a nurse . . .

Following my retirement, I had the time to embark on a UK tour to talk about Mary Seacole and help raise urgently needed funds for her memorial statue. Fortunately, invitations to speak came from a wide variety of individuals and organisations, including nurses, trade unions, Black and minority associations and women's groups. They were wonderful sessions that demonstrated the appeal of Mary to so many people, and from such a wide range of backgrounds. This positive response refuted critics who dismissed the idea that 'Mother Seacole' could ever be considered as a role model.

The audiences well and truly understood that the statue campaign wasn't about undermining the achievements of Florence Nightingale – but they did want to hear about other historical nursing figures too, as articulated by Felicia, a director of nursing: 'We were always brought up with Florence Nightingale. That's all we knew. We never had any Black, Asian or Chinese nursing figures that we could aspire to. I had never learned about Mary Seacole – didn't have a clue before I met you.'

I really wish that we could be taught about the achievements of other Crimean War nurses alongside Florence Nightingale and Mary Seacole. There were many, but examples include Betsi Cadwaladr from Wales, Eliza Mackenzie (a naval nurse) from Scotland and the Irish Sisters of Mercy under Mother Francis Bridgeman. There was also the Russian nurse Darya Lavrentyevna Mikhailova, otherwise known as 'Dasha of Sevastopol'.[5]

My talks about Mary Seacole continued for an extended period of time, as it took the charity over twelve long years to raise the original target of half a million pounds (which was quite depressing at times, but the encouragement of friends kept my spirits up – such as my friend Joan B's wonderful comment: 'You follow through with everything, so for me the Mary Seacole statue will happen. You are Mary Seacole!'). Then came a last-minute additional and unexpectedly hefty charge from the construction company to instal the memorial. Happily, the money was secured in November 2015 from Her Majesty's Treasury, courtesy of funds allocated to charities from banking fines.

The wonderful memorial statue was unveiled by Baroness Floella Benjamin on 30 June 2016 in the gardens of St Thomas' Hospital, overlooking the River Thames and the Houses of Parliament. I attended with both Azuka and my granddaughter, Rhianne, who was eight at the time. Remarkably, it is the first one named for a Black woman in the UK; I see her now, striding forwards, and think she's keeping an eye on the politicians. For groups of people who don't always feel accepted, it's so important to see her. For my granddaughter to see someone who looks like her, with Black skin – it brought such joy to my heart.

The ceremony proved to be incredibly inspiring. While the previous few days had been cold and wet, the sun decided to shine for a few hours and provided some Jamaican weather for the near 400 invited guests. Reporter Sir William Howard Russell would be delighted, having written this about Mary Seacole in 1857: 'I trust that England will not forget one who nursed her sick, who sought out her wounded to aid and succour them, and who performed the last offices for some of her illustrious dead.'

A couple of weeks later, Rhianne came to stay with me during the summer holidays. We had a lovely day exploring London and going on the London Eye. I said to her: 'Is there anything else you'd like to do?' She looked up at me and said: 'Please could we go see Mary?'

Chapter 41:

Becoming Dame Elizabeth Nneka Anionwu

In November 2016, a letter dropped through my door containing an invitation for me to accept a damehood in the 2017 New Year's Honours list. I had to read it three times – once again, it was for services to nursing, but also to the Mary Seacole Statue Appeal, and I thought, 'Ooh that's all right.' I was so surprised and confused, because I thought I was too much of an awkward customer to receive such a senior honour (and having already received a CBE in 2001).

As I'd previously done, I talked it over with a trusted friend, who wouldn't leak the confidential news. The friend I spoke to said I should accept it for two reasons: one, because of the whole issue of Black nurses in the NHS and their low status – in 2019, only eight of the 231 NHS trusts in England had a chief nurse from a Black and minority ethnic (BME) background – and two, because of the feel-good factor it would generate.[1]

When I started dealing with nursing issues (such as sickle cell and thalassaemia) at a national level, I was challenging policy, but there were several chief nursing officers who made it clear to me that they never took it personally. What I was saying was needed, and they found it helpful when people not only challenged existing policy and practice, but who also gave suggestions of solutions. I wasn't aware of how people at the top get fed information about what's taking place on the ground, so it was enlightening to know they were paying attention.

Even now, I'm still in two minds about the awards system – and I don't judge anyone for turning them down – but after accepting the damehood, I witnessed the impact of it on the nursing profession, particularly the pride of Black nurses and midwives. It gives them confidence to see that people who look like them, who are doing similar work to them and who historically haven't been recognised are now getting the honours they deserve. Previously, it's been the Establishment who have nominated and received the titles, but this is changing and anyone can now put someone forward for an honour.

So on February 2017, during a huge storm, I travelled to Buckingham Palace to receive my damehood from Queen Elizabeth II with Azuka, Rhianne and my cousin-in-law Elaine. It was very exciting, but I was extremely nervous because I was the second in line to receive an award, after the politician Shirley Williams, who was appointed to the Order of the Companions of Honour for 'services to political and public life' (Rhianne presumed she was the Queen). As I went to accept my damehood, the Queen asked me about sickle cell and Mary Seacole – she said she'd recently met the Jamaican High Commissioner who had said how pleased he was that the statue was sited in London.

Then, in 2019, I was presented with a Lifetime Achievement Award at the Pride of Britain Awards, which celebrate 'truly remarkable people'. I was sitting at home listening to the radio, when I got the surprise call telling me, 'You've won, and you've won the major award of 2019.' On the night, I was standing on the stage talking to the host, Carol Vorderman, when she announced, 'and to present the award is Janet Jackson . . .' Seeing Miss Jackson slinking across the stage was wonderful.

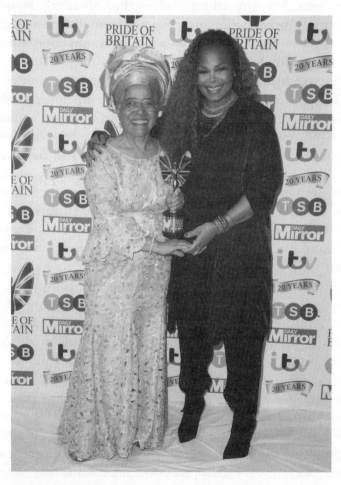

Me with Janet Jackson at the Pride of Britain Awards, 2019.

In this same year, I also received four honorary doctorate awards from the University of St Andrews, Brunel University London, Birmingham City University and the University of Manchester. The award from Birmingham City University was fittingly presented by its chancellor, Sir Lenny Henry, who I'd worked with when he was a patron of the Sickle Cell Society and had made an appeal on Radio 4 on behalf of the charity. Similarly, Lemn Sissay, chancellor of the University of Manchester, was a welcome connection to Jessica Huntley, as Bogle-L'Ouverture published some of his early work.

One person who didn't get to see me receive these honours was my mother, who died in 2003. Ken had died in August 1994 aged sixty-eight, following a stroke, and it was the only funeral where I haven't felt any sense of grief for the deceased person; I shed absolutely no tears at the service. However, it was wonderful that Mum, Mick, Frank, Marion, Pam and I were all together; it had been such a long time since it had happened.

Following Ken's death, Pam and her husband bought a house with a granny flat attached for my mother. This was such a kind and generous gesture, as it provided Mum with security, close to her family and grandchildren. She was able to spend the remaining nine years of her life there, very content with all of her activities. Aside from her family, she would read, walk her dog, learn new languages such as Russian and watch wildlife documentaries. She wrote to me saying: 'I joined Mensa in 1979 and found their activities (or such of their many and varied activities as I was able to take part in) very stimulating. I tried my hand at writing for some of their publications and had a number of poems and short articles printed.'

Religion also played an important role, and Mum became involved with the Methodists. Writing to me on 8 April 1994, just four months before Ken's death, she reflected: 'Looking back over the ups and downs, in my own small way I can say with the Psalmist, "Thou hast brought me to great honour and comforted me on every side." May He do the same in His goodness for all my children.' She eventually switched to the Church of England, where she could take the sacrament. As she explained: 'No account of my life would be complete, however, without mentioning that during this period, God led me to make a serious study of the Scriptures, and to turn to Him in prayer and meditation. Even from the first stirrings of this conversion experience, life seemed to become easier to cope with.'

When Azuka and I saw Mum in September 2003, she seemed well but she did tell me of being scared that she was going to die. Weeks later, Marion and Pam called me to say she was extremely unwell and hardly eating or drinking. It turned out to be the opportunity to nurse my mother in her final illness.

In January 2004, I described the experience in a *Nursing Times* column:

When she suddenly deteriorated, I set off on the motorway from London with a heavy heart. I was shocked by how frail and bedridden she had become and, as the only nurse in the family, I was aware that my sisters were looking to me for guidance. I was somewhat taken aback that part of me wished that I did not have any nursing knowledge, because it meant that I understood that she was extremely ill.

However, it was with great satisfaction that I was able

to give her a bed bath, ably helped by my sisters. At this point I was delighted to be a nurse. The opportunity to make her feel more comfortable and assist her to take a small amount of fluids was both gratifying and extremely consoling. Her senses were still intact because, as soon as I had left, she told one of my sisters that my visit had turned out to be a busman's holiday.

A few days later, on 27 October, Mum died at home in the early hours of the morning, aged seventy-seven. Cause of death was bronchopneumonia, congestive cardiac failure, hypertension and chronic renal impairment.

The funeral demonstrated the love of all of her children, as Mick, Frank, Marion, Pam and I assembled to mourn her loss. We were the ones she had fought so hard to protect, and to ensure that we had a decent life. It was a very difficult ceremony for everyone. While crying for the suffering Mum had endured, I knew that she would have been happy that we were all together and celebrating her life. Uncle Michael and Auntie Pat also attended, which enabled Mick, Frank, Marion and Pam to meet them at last. Sadly, transport difficulties made it impossible for my Auntie Sheila to attend. My paternal cousin-in-law Elaine recalled: 'When I went to your mother's funeral in 2003, I did wonder how it would be for you. I hadn't seen that side of the family around you before, but they just took you in. I had the feeling that they thought they had to protect you a bit, you know, the sadness, and Azuka was there with them.'

It is ironic that although she had so much less to leave than Dad, Mum was more organised. She left a will and had already paid for her funeral expenses. There was £66.44 in her savings account. It was in stark contrast to my wealthier barrister father, who died intestate.

Most importantly, her presence was always there in the background, constantly loving and worrying about all five of her children. Mum's greatest joy was to be with her children and she was loved by all of us. Frank's view was that 'Mum had inner strength and there wasn't an ounce of wrong in her.' Mick, her eldest son, would die in 2015 aged sixty-one, so she never suffered the anguish of losing him. Mum always wished she could have helped us more, but we had in fact been supported by her in so many ways.

Chapter 42:

Dreams from My Mother

All the achievements I'm so proud of – being the UK's first sickle cell specialist nurse; overcoming discrimination – getting into nursing in the first place and qualifying as a health visitor, despite the obstacles placed in my way; setting up the Mary Seacole Centre for Nursing Practice, which had a huge impact during a time when there were no widespread resources; and getting a PhD, even though it took forever – have all been inspired by a multi-ethnic perspective, because that's who I am.

Currently, the country is dealing with Covid-19, which is a dreadful illness for everybody. It's incredibly contagious, but figures show that it has had a disproportionate impact on my Black and minority ethnic colleagues: Black people are four times more likely to die from Covid-19 than white people; and, despite accounting for just 20 per cent of the NHS workforce (44 per cent among medics), 94 per cent of doctors and 71 per cent of nurses who have died were Black, Asian or minority ethnic.[1]

Looking at the case of someone like twenty-eight-year-old nurse Mary Agyeiwaa Agyapong, who died after giving birth at Luton and Dunstable Hospital, where she also worked, shows up a lot of the issues surrounding these figures. In an inquest into her death, testimonies showed that she felt 'pressured to work' and was discharged despite her own reservations.[2] It proves that people feel like they don't have the power or authority to say no to being exposed on the frontline to a higher viral load of Covid-19.

Often, people from Black and minority ethnic backgrounds are dependent on work because of where they are in society. They have to earn money – like many others, obviously – but quite a few aren't in a position to argue with their managers; and the higher up the NHS you go, the lower the proportion there are of people from these backgrounds.

If staff don't have the clout to say they're vulnerable because they're the breadwinners and desperately need a job, they're not going to argue with the boss, are they? Especially with all the unemployment Covid-19 has caused, because you can easily be replaced. It's the fear of being sacked, the fear of unemployment, the fear of poverty, never mind the fear of the wretched illness itself. Plus, they might be experiencing the added trauma of witnessing illness and death among their family and local community.

We know that Covid-19 is incredibly transmissible, so you are particularly vulnerable if you live in overcrowded situations and are someone who cannot work from home, especially if you are employed in a factory or organisation that hasn't taken precautions for their staff or where personal protective equipment (PPE) hasn't been issued or doesn't meet the right standard of quality. It is absolutely obvious that the illness is going to spread rapidly through the vulnerable workforce. Reading the 2021 Commission on Race and Ethnic Disparities, which was set up by the government in response to the Black Lives Matter protests of 2020, the denial that there's any institutional racism in the UK is utterly astounding.

As Toni Morrison said in a 1975 speech at Portland State Black Studies Center in Oregon, USA:

> The function, the very serious function of racism, is distraction. It keeps you from doing your work. It keeps you explaining, over and over again, your reason for being. Somebody says you have no language and you spend twenty years proving that you do. Somebody says your head isn't shaped properly so you have scientists working on the fact that it is. Somebody says you have no art, so you dredge that up. Somebody says you have no kingdoms, so you dredge that up. None of this is necessary. There will always be one more thing.

Looking at the anti-vaccination movement, it's people of all backgrounds and classes, but they are united by not trusting the state for whatever reason. The mistrust that Black people have towards the state has been caused by historic events. For example, the New Cross fire in 1981, which killed thirteen young Black people, led to the Black People's Day of Action because the police quickly dropped an investigation into a possible racist attack, instead apportioning blame to the teenagers themselves.

Similarly in healthcare, Depo-Provera, the contraceptive injection, was tested on human beings using a disproportionate number of African-American women and low-income European American women from 1967 to 1978.[3] There's the fact that Black women are four times more likely to die from complications surrounding pregnancy and childbirth or that Black people are more than four times as likely as white people to be detained under the Mental Health Act.[4] What Covid-19 has done is to expose existing health inequalities.

Stigma was an important issue that came to the surface in my conversations about sickle cell in the 1970s. People were wary of talking about the condition because it was seen as a Black issue (the National Front used it in their propaganda) and they were worried about being seen as a burden on the NHS or British state. Meanwhile, families from the Caribbean were asking me, 'Why haven't we heard about this before now? It must be a conspiracy.' This is an example of how people can be made to feel inferior because of their ethnicity and the conditions they are more likely to experience.

While encouraging progress has been made in the care of those affected by sickle cell disease, there is absolutely no room for complacency. This was tragically demonstrated in April 2021 with the circumstances surrounding the death in 2019 of Evan Nathan Smith in a north London hospital – he had dialled 999 from his hospital bed after being refused oxygen.[5] An inquest concluded: 'There was a failure to appreciate the significance of those symptoms by those looking after Mr Smith at the time.'

It is clear to me now that I have carried a bellyful of anger throughout my life. It's why I've done what I've done, fortunately using the energy of that anger in a positive rather than a negative way. Otherwise, it could have led to the kind of depression that forces you to retreat under the duvet, blaming yourself and cutting yourself off from resources that could be of help. Reading Barack Obama's *Dreams from My Father*, as he gradually started to realise the impact of race, I also slowly began to understand my own deep-seated rage, and how it has driven me to fight against racism, injustice and health inequalities. I'm a relatively stable person who relates well to people from different backgrounds and positions of authority, who makes friends easily and who is intelligent. All these factors have helped me to progress. However, what has driven me into the areas I specialise in is anger.

On reflection, I can appreciate the multiple factors that have influenced my attitudes, behaviour and political activism. They include having been in care, being 'illegitimate', living in poverty, suffering physical abuse, being mixed-race, being a woman and being a single mother. It doesn't make sense to my logical way of thinking if someone thinks a person is inferior just because of their background or skin colour. If there's a gap in services here or hatred shown to a person there, that's what gets me worked up. But you can't achieve everything you want by becoming a raging bull continually crashing into a china shop. I can see people's fear sometimes when I go off on one and sometimes I quite enjoy it, but I have also realised when to rein it in. Tackling sickle cell disease was a big learning experience; it taught me how to argue confidently with policy-makers and health providers when their justification for inadequate resources was, 'Oh it's a minority issue.'

To fight back, I had to get the facts by speaking to people who were affected by the condition and pulling those narratives together, then working with them to build their confidence so they could tell their own stories. I started to see the effect all this was having on others and that gave me confidence. I watched other people to see how they were achieving change – for example, in the 1980s, when the gay community came together across classes and ethnicities to combat Aids and HIV. These activists had so much rage, because there were drugs that could save people but the Reagan administration in the US didn't want to even mention the problem; the way they used media, music and entertainment to pressure the state was huge.[6]

Going to the US in the late 1970s and seeing the work on sickle cell there made me realise I could make a personal difference, too. Meeting specialist sickle cell nurses in Los Angeles and San Francisco made me understand that it wasn't just about campaigning but that, as a nurse myself, I could physically make a change to people's lives. In those six years, when I was the only specialist sickle cell nurse at Brent, I also realised the power of public speaking. I had to respond to countrywide requests to explain what we were doing and I watched the Brent model begin to spread across the UK as a result. People would contact me about the obstacles and challenges they were facing, and I was able to advise and help them to find solutions. Who should they link with? How could they obtain funding? Like Black Lives Matter and US voting rights activist Stacey Abrams, this community development action (which was seen as a radical term by the Health Education Council and banned at one point) was a grassroots bottom-up approach.

Representation is a human rights issue. People should have the opportunity to progress in their career, regardless of their skin colour or background. There's also a common sense aspect to having a more representative group of people within all the levels of your organisation. If a diverse group can input ideas from their own life experiences, you will have a richer awareness of the needs that the organisation should be addressing. Sections within society need to see themselves represented and their needs being addressed. If only the needs of those in power are being addressed, then it causes tension, anger and depression. Everyone wants to feel valued – even if they don't want to progress up the ladder, they need to know that, if they fulfil the criteria, there's nothing stopping them.

People also need to develop that inner confidence and not absorb all the negativity around them; you can do this by reading and engaging in discourse. I also say, be aware that there may be surprising people who may want to support you; it might even be that white senior male, so keep your eyes open. I've had many different people see something in me, including the medical officer who encouraged me to apply for nursing when I was a vulnerable teenager; Jessica Huntley, who introduced me to and involved me in so many Black campaigning events; Dr Brozović, who recognised my huge interest in sickle cell and encouraged my confidence to ask questions and write articles; Professor Akinyanju, who involved me with educational courses in Nigeria and while I was struggling to complete my PhD thesis told me to take six months off when I was too frightened to ask; my PhD supervisor, Alan Beattie, who took exceptional measures to get me into the academic environment even when I didn't have the relevant qualifications – he could see I could do a PhD way before I could – and Professor Marcus Pembrey, who opened that academic door for me when I was going to return to health visiting. Then there was Dorothy Boswell, a tough cookie and the CEO of the US National Association for Sickle Cell Disease, who supported my efforts back in the UK.

One of the ways I've tried to give back is by being available to go and talk to Black nurses and midwives and the voluntary sector. From the title of my talk, 'From Sickle to Seacole', people can see positive outcomes from the campaigns I've been involved with. Nowadays, I talk about 'getting on, despite the odds', which appeals to people who feel they're being trampled on, who can't achieve, and not through lack of trying. What does my life show them? Hopefully, the varied obstacles I've overcome. Feedback includes liking that I can stand on stage and say things people don't expect me to say. I'm retired, so not accountable to anybody. When people freely discuss their racist experiences within the NHS, my response is, 'Get the evidence. Why do you think it's racist? Are you a member of a trade union? You don't need to fight this alone.' Adopt the belief: 'Don't let them grind you down.'

I also know that when I get overwhelmed with issues, it's important to have coping strategies. I call it my toolbox: such as talking to a friend or relative, going for a walk, watching comedy on television or dancing to music. My favourite thing to put on at the moment is the reggae album *Blackheart Man* by Bunny Wailer, who died in 2021. I put my playlist on shuffle when I go for walks and it's a mixture of classical, highlife, reggae and Irish folk music, plus songs from beautiful voices such as Kathleen Ferrier and Paul Robeson. It leaves me calmed and uplifted.

Music is a connection to the cultural heritage of both of my parents – who also gave me intelligence and logic (after all, my father was a barrister). They both accepted me in their own ways: my dad with love and support, and my mum with love and courage. Thinking about that time just after the Second World War, when people like me were rare and my mother wasn't even married – she didn't give into the pressure to have me adopted, and that obstinacy was down to love. This, during a time when the pressure of family and society were so overwhelming that women were forced to give up their children even if they didn't want to. My friend Nina reflected: 'I don't know where you get your strength from, but you are very resilient. You are mindful of whatever things are happening and you bounce back stronger. Maybe it's from your mother, because she's probably had to put up with much more than your father did.'

I think about what my grandparents, mother and father would have made of my damehood, achievements and awards. From the perspective of an Irish immigrant family and from that of my dad – who, while part of the Establishment, was still a product of colonisation – they would have been so proud. My grandfather had such pride in his daughter's success and, thinking about the expression, 'The apple never falls far from the tree,' he and my grandmother would have taken great joy in my achievements. I know my auntie Pat is very proud. And despite all the shock, horror, stigma and suffering surrounding my birth, it turned out well for me in the end.

Seventy plus years later, being mixed-race goes virtually without comment. Nearly, but not quite: think about a senior member of the Royal Family questioning how dark Archie's skin colour might be when he was born, or the derisive comments aimed at Barack Obama ('He's not really American') and Mary Seacole ('She's not really Black').[7] There's been such a huge change in demographics and mixed-race people are now the fastest-growing ethnic group in the UK; it's here, whether people like it or not.

My friend Mia described me in her own inimitable way: 'I've seen you as a light-skinned Black person. It was only later on when you started talking about your memories of growing up that I realised you were mixed-race. Identity has always been an issue that comes up in the community, particularly for mixed-race people. It's very important for them that they talk about their identity. You don't ram it down people's throats.'

Now, I feel utterly at ease and proud of who I am. I tell

my daughter and granddaughter that people judging you for your skin colour is their problem. I instil confidence and pride in them, offering advice and support if they ever want it. I didn't originally have that family role model in terms of skin colour. The most important thing is that, internally, you are at ease with how you look and who you are. You can deal with stigma better when you realise that people have no reason to think less of you – it's only a desire to make you feel inferior. I know that my daughter has learned and observed from me, and my granddaughter has learned from her mother and me.

At my seventieth birthday, Rhianne composed and read out a poem called 'My Grandma':

If someone asks me who is the most amazing, special, kind grandma, I'd say you. You are so special to me because . . .
You make me your special porridge, to be fair it is better than my mummy's porridge!
You make me laugh, ha, ha, ha
You buy me books with powerful women in!
You're like a girl version of Jeremy Corbyn because you are strong, kind and care for people that need it.
You buy me dolls with skin and hair like mine and it fills me with so much joy!
I love you, Grandma, I could never ask for a better grandma than you!!!

My mother's dreams were family and career. She didn't get to fulfil her career, but I have. When people learn about my mum's life, there's a natural sadness that she didn't get to achieve her academic potential and, yes, it is a shame, but all five children were so close to her throughout her life. If I could say one thing to my mother, it would be thank you.

Thank you for giving up your dreams of studying at Cambridge, and thank you for your courage and withstanding the pain in order to make a home for me.

Her continued presence in my life and what she had to overcome for me can never be underestimated. She also knew when to ask for help, contacting my grandparents to take me in when it must have been very, very difficult. It's taught me to ask for help when I need it, too. She had her religion and, while I don't subscribe to that, I do have faith. Faith in people and in the fact that the goodness in enough individuals can outweigh the evil that exists in the world. I've been on the receiving end of such kindness and friendship – it has and still does help me enormously.

What fascinates me about my mother is that despite her incredible intellectual ability, it's the pride and what she gave up for her children that's extraordinary. My sister Marion explained to me how Mum and I were so alike: 'Mum thought the world of you; she loved us all the same. You are similar to her more than anything, not only with your intelligence, but also your determination. Mum had quiet determination. You're a much more forceful character and you've been able to perhaps achieve all the things that she couldn't. You've led the life that Mum should have also led.'

Acknowledgements

All of the following people have been extremely helpful to me during the process of producing these memoirs. Many kindly agreed to be interviewed, and my thanks go to Nalini Patel for transcribing the interviews and to all those who have provided assistance in numerous other ways. I am extremely grateful to you all and apologise for any omissions.

Dr Elizabeth Dormandy has been an incredibly supportive and critical friend to me throughout the entire writing of this book. Our regular meetings and lunches at Friends House in London made all the hard work that much more enjoyable!

Also, huge thanks to Catherine Gough of Fine Words for a wonderfully calm approach and for her expert and speedy editing.

Now to all of my Furlong and Anionwu family members in the UK, Nigeria and the USA! You have really gone out of your way to help me, and I have really appreciated all the support and enthusiasm from so many relatives. They include aunts Pat Glass, Doreen Furlong and Nwachinemelu Joy Anionwu; sisters Marion and Pam, brother Frank; cousins Chinyelugo Osita Anionwu, Ugobueze Joy Ikeme Arah, Dave Glass, Anne Kearsley and Elaine Unegbu.

My appreciation to all of my lovely friends for all the information and advice provided: Akunne Abadom and family, Akunnia Ejor Abomile and family, Juliet Alexander, Suzette Alleyne, Professor Karl Atkin, Dr Carol Barton, Alan Beattie, Ann Clwyd MP, Dr Moira Dick, Sandra Edwards, Franca

Egbuche, Rose Grant, Jean Gray, Dada Imarogbe, Professor Baba Inusa, Wendy Irwin, John James OBE, Ursula Johnson, Mariama Kabba, Felicia Kwaku OBE, Marvlyn Le Fleurier, Sarah Massengale-Gregg, Dr Alison May, Mia Morris OBE, Joan Myers OBE, Freddie Onyechi, Nina Patel, Professor Marcus Pembrey, Michelle Pickard, Sue Rees, Joan Saddler OBE, Paelo Saddler, Ramesh Seewoodhary, Janet Shea-Simonds, Megan Thomas, Jackie Wetherill and Alison Winter.

A special thank you to the late John Roberts CBE, QC for finding my father. Also to Siobhán Clemons, Team Leader – Origins Service, Father Hudson's Care for her sensitive and helpfulmanner in responding to my enquiries.

Ben Galley, publishing consultant at Shelf Help, is greatly appreciated for all his helpful advice.

My thanks also to professional genealogists Megan Owens and Records Ireland, Irish Family History Research Service together with Wolverhampton Archives and Local Studies.

I am also very grateful to Malorie Blackman OBE, writer and former Children's Laureate for her wonderful foreword to this book.

Professor Jane Cummings CBE, former Chief Nursing Officer for England, and Conrad Bryan, Trustee, the Association of Mixed Race Irish, kindly set aside time to read my memoirs and provided extremely positive feedback – their quotes have been hugely appreciated!

I would like to thank Francesca Brown and all at Orion who have helped in the publishing of this revised and updated edition of my original self-published memoir, especially Sam Eades, Zoe Yang, Jo Whitford, Elizabeth Allen, Yadira Da Trindade, Paul Stark and Debbie Holmes.

Finally, a very special word of thanks to my daughter, Azuka, and granddaughter, Rhianne, for their constant love and encouragement.

CREDITS

Seven Dials would like to thank everyone at Orion who worked on the publication of *Dreams from My Mother*:

Editor
Sam Eades
Zoe Yang

Copy-editor
Natasha Onwuemezi

Proofreader
Claire Dean

Editorial Management
Jo Whitford
Charlie Panayiotou
Jane Hughes
Claire Boyle
Jake Alderson

Audio
Paul Stark
Amber Bates

Contracts
Anne Goddard
Paul Bulos

Design
Debbie Holmes
Joanna Ridley
Nick May
Clare Sivell
Helen Ewing
Natalie Dawkins

Finance
Jennifer Muchan
Jasdip Nandra
Rabale Mustafa
Ibukun Ademefun
Levancia Clarendon
Tom Costello

Marketing
Yadira Da Trindade

Production
Claire Keep
Fiona McIntosh

Publicity
Elizabeth Allen

Sales

Jen Wilson
Victoria Laws
Esther Waters
Lucy Brem
Frances Doyle
Ben Goddard
Georgina Cutler
Jack Hallam
Ellie Kyrke-Smith
Inês Figuiera
Barbara Ronan
Andrew Hally
Dominic Smith
Deborah Deyong
Lauren Buck
Maggy Park
Linda McGregor
Sinead White
Jemimah James
Rachael Jones
Jack Dennison
Nigel Andrews
Ian Williamson
Julia Benson
Declan Kyle
Robert Mackenzie
Imogen Clarke
Megan Smith
Charlotte Clay
Rebecca Cobbold

Operations

Jo Jacobs
Sharon Willis
Lisa Pryde

Rights

Susan Howe
Richard King
Krystyna Kujawinska
Jessica Purdue
Louise Henderson

Picture Credits

All images are from the author's personal collection, except for the following:

INTEGRATED IMAGES

p.58: Reproduced by kind permission of Ann Ellis
p.307: © Alamy

Suggested Reading

Achebe, Chinua. *Things Fall Apart*. London: Heinemann, 1962.
— *A Man of the People*. London: Heinemann, 1966.
— *There Was a Country: A Personal History of Biafra*. London: Allen Lane, 2012.

Bland, Lucy. *Britain's 'Brown Babies': The Stories of Children Born to Black GIs and White Women in the Second World War*. Manchester: Manchester University Press, 2019.

Coard, Bernard. *How the West Indian Child Is Made Educationally Subnormal in the British School System*. London: New Beacon Books, 1971.

Davis, Angela. *Angela Davis: An Autobiography*. London: Hutchinson, 1975.

De St. Jorre, John. *The Nigerian Civil War*. London: Hodder & Stoughton, 1972.

Eldridge, Cleaver. *Soul on Ice*. New York City, NY: McGraw-Hill 1968.

Fanon, Frantz. *Black Skin, White Masks*. London: MacGibbon & Kee, 1968.

Jackson, George. *Soledad Brother: The Prison Letters of George Jackson*. London: Penguin, 1973.

Nwapa, Flora. *Efuru*. London: Heinemann, 1966.

Obama, Barack. *Dreams from My Father*. Edinburgh: Canongate, 2007.

Roberts, Pamela. *Black Oxford: The Untold Stories of Oxford University's Black Scholars*. Oxford: Signal Books, 2013.

Robeson, Paul. *Here I Stand*. New York City, NY: Othello Associates, 1958.

Rodney, Walter. *How Europe Underdeveloped Africa*. London: Bogle-L'Ouverture, 1972.

Safo, Lucy. *Cry a Whisper*. London: Bogle-L'Ouverture Press, 1993.

Seacole, Mary. *Wonderful Adventures of Mrs Seacole in Many Lands*. London: James Blackwood, 1857.

Selvon, Samuel, *The Lonely Londoners*. London: Allan Wingate, 1956.

Soyinka, Wole. *The Man Died: Prison Notes of Wole Soyinka*. London: Rex Collings, 1972.

Tressell, Robert. *The Ragged Trousered Philanthropists*. London: Grant Richards Ltd, 1914.

Zobel, Joseph. *Black Shack Alley*. Boulder, CO: Lynne Rienner Publishers, Inc., 1980.

Endnotes

2. Cambridge Life

1. 'The Rising Tide: Women at Cambridge', Stuart Roberts, University of Cambridge, undated. https://www.cam.ac.uk/TheRisingTide [Accessed: 31 March 2021].
2. 'Turned away at the gates: the struggle for places for women at Cambridge', Shannon Rawlins, Varsity, 15 March 2019. https://www.varsity.co.uk/features/17317 [Accessed: 31 March 2021].

3. The Dossier

1. 'The Rise and Fall of the Workhouse', Charlotte Hodgman, History Extra, 25 April 2021 (originally published in the *BBC History Magazine*, 20 December 2010). https://www.historyextra.com/period/victorian/the-rise-and-fall-of-the-workhouse/ [Accessed: 11 May 2021].
2. J. Robinson, *In the Family Way: Illegitimacy Between the Great War and the Swinging Sixties* (Viking, 2015).
3. 'Child Migration Programmes Investigation Report', Independent Inquiry: Child Sexual Abuse, March 2018. https://www.iicsa.org.uk/publications/investigation/child-migration/part-c-detailed-examination-institutional-responses/sending-institutions/210-father-hudsons [Accessed: 31 March 2021].

4. Uncovering History

1. 'Number of Live births in the United Kingdom (UK) from 1931 to 1960', Statista Research Department, 28 August 2013. https://www.statista.com/statistics/281965/live-births-in-the-united-kingdom-uk-1931-1960/ [Accessed: 31 March 2021].

2. 'The Catholic church sold my child', Martin Sixsmith, *Guardian*, 19 September 2009. https://www.theguardian.com/lifeandstyle/2009/sep/19/catholic-church-sold-child [Accessed: 31 March 2021].

3. 'Rationing', Bodmin Keep: Cornwall's Army Museum, April 2020. https://bodminkeep.org/wp-content/uploads/2020/04/KEEP-KIDS_Rationing_Issue_1_April_2020_-1.pdf [Accessed: 31 March 2021].

5. Hard Times

1. 'Review of Jacqueline Jenkinson, *Black 1919: Riots, Racism and Resistance in Imperial Britain*', Dr Laura Tabili, Reviews in History (840), December 2009, https://reviews.history.ac.uk/review/840, quoted in 'Black British people', Wikipedia, footnote 146. https://en.wikipedia.org/wiki/Black_British_people [Accessed: 31 March 2021].

2. D. Olusoga, *Black and British: A Forgotten History* (Macmillan, 2016).

3. L. Bland, *Britain's 'Brown Babies': The Stories of Children Born to Black GIs and White Women in the Second World War* (Manchester University Press, 2019), p.34.

6. Mother and Baby

1. 'Maternal Care and Mental Health', John Bowlby, World Health Organization (1951). https://pages.uoregon.edu/eherman/teaching/texts/Bowlby%20Maternal%20Care%20and%20Mental%20Health.pdf [Accessed: 31 March 2021].

2. 'The life-long prisoners of State-funded, church-run institutions', Sinead Pembroke, *Irish Times*, 8 March 2017. https://www.irishtimes.com/opinion/the-life-long-prisoners-of-state-funded-church-run-institutions-1.3001635 [Accessed: 31 March 2021].

11. Future Foundations

1. J. Kelly, *Rock Me Gently: A Memoir of a Convent Childhood* (Bloomsbury, 2006).

2. Scottish Child Abuse Inquiry, 'Sisters of Nazareth Press Release', 11 December 2019. https://www.childabuseinquiry.scot/news/ sisters-of-nazareth-press-release/ [Accessed: 31 March 2021].
3. B. Adams, *Pater Noster* (Lulu.com, 2007).
4. 'Britain's child migrant programme: why 130,000 children were shipped abroad', Caroline Davies, *Guardian*, 27 February 2017. https://www.theguardian.com/society/2017/feb/27/ britains-child-migrant-programme-why-130000-children-were-shipped-abroad [Accessed: 31 March 2021].
5. 'Child Migration Programmes Investigation Report', Independent Inquiry: Child Sexual Abuse, March 2018. https:// www.iicsa.org.uk/publications/investigation/child-migration/ part-c-detailed-examination-institutional-responses/send-ing-institutions/210-father-hudsons [Accessed: 31 March 2021].
6. 'Raymond Brand', Australian National Maritime Museum, undated. https://www.sea.museum/explore/online-exhibi-tions/britains-child-migrants/new-lands-new-life/schemes-dig-in/raymond-brand [Accessed: 11 May 2021].

12. Mum and Ken

1. 'Prescription Charges', Socialist Health Association, undated. https://www.sochealth.co.uk/national-health-service/access-to-health-care-and-charges/prescription-charges/ [Accessed: 31 March 2021].

17. Sudden Departure

1. 'The story of black nurses in the UK didn't start with Windrush', Lynn Eaton, *Guardian*, 13 May 2020. https://www.theguardian. com/society/2020/may/13/black-nurses-in-uk-didnt-start-with-windrush-covid-19-deaths [Accessed: 1 April 2021].

21. New Horizons

1. R. Bunce and P. Field, *Darcus Howe. A Political Biography* (Bloomsbury, 2014).

24. A Radical Health Visitor

1. 'East African Asians', Minority Rights Group International, undated. https://minorityrights.org/minorities/east-african-asians/ [Accessed: 31 March 2021].

2. Commonwealth Immigrants Act 1968.

3. 'Expulsion of Asians from Uganda', Wikipedia, undated. https://en.wikipedia.org/wiki/Expulsion_of_Asians_from_Uganda [Accessed: 31 March 2021]; '1972: Expelled Ugandans arrive in UK', BBC On This Day, 18 September 2015. http://news.bbc.co.uk/onthisday/hi/dates/stories/september/18/newsid_2522000/2522627.stm [Accessed: 31 March 2021].

4. 'The day Britain took in 27,000 refugees', Jon Snow, Channel 4 News, 6 September 2015. https://www.channel4.com/news/by/jon-snow/blogs/day-britain-27000-refugees [Accessed: 31 March 2021]; 'They fled with nothing but built a new empire', *Guardian*, 11 August 2002. https://www.theguardian.com/uk/2002/aug/11/race.world [Accessed: 31 March 2021]

5. 'Eric and Jessica Huntley', Black History Month, 25 August 2015. https://www.blackhistorymonth.org.uk/article/gallery/test-diane-julie-abbott-politician/ [Accessed: 31 March 2021].

6. 'Forty years of *How Europe Underdeveloped Africa*', Nigel Westmaas, Climate & Capitalism, 27 June 2012. https://climateandcapitalism.com/2012/06/27/forty-years-of-how-europe-underdeveloped-africa/ [Accessed: 31 March 2021].

25. Speaking Out

1. M. Hickman et al. (1999), 'Mapping the prevalence of sickle cell and beta thalassaemia in England: estimating and validating ethnic-specific rates', *British Journal of Haematology*, 104: 860–867. https://doi.org/10.1046/j.1365-2141.1999.01275.x [Accessed: 2 April 2021].

2. Graham R. Serjeant and Beryl E. Serjeant, *Sickle Cell Disease* (Oxford University Press, 2001).

3. 'Overview: sickle cell disease', NHS, undated.

https://www.nhs.uk/conditions/sickle-cell-disease/ [Accessed: 10 April 2021]; 'Overview: thalassaemia', NHS, undated. https://www.nhs.uk/conditions/thalassaemia/ [Accessed: 10 April 2021].

4. 'Overview: cystic fibrosis', NHS, undated. https://www.nhs.uk/conditions/cystic-fibrosis/ [Accessed: 2 April 2021]; 'NHS Screening Programmes in England', Public Health England, March 2019. https://assets.publishing.service.gov.uk/government/uploads/system/uploads/attachment_data/file/783537/NHS_Screening_Programmes_in_England_2017_to_2018_final.pdf [Accessed: 2 April 2021].

5. S. Claster and E. P. Vichinsky (2003), 'Managing Sickle Cell Disease', *BMJ*, 337 (7424): 1151–5.

26. Breaking Out

1. 'Black Panther Party', Wikipedia, undated. https://en.wikipedia.org/wiki/Black_Panther_Party [Accessed: 31 March 2021].

2. 'March on Washington', History, 29 October 2009, updated 16 March 2021. https://www.history.com/topics/black-history/march-on-washington [Accessed: 31 March 2021].

3. 'The Notting Hill riots of 1958', Warwick University, last revised 11 March 2020. https://warwick.ac.uk/services/library/mrc/studying/docs/racism/riots [Accessed: 31 March 2021].

4. 'Advocates of Bussing Should Learn from British History and Not Just the US', Vicki Butler, The Huffington Post, 4 October 2012, updated 4 December 2012. https://www.huffingtonpost.co.uk/vicki-butler/bussing-uk-segregation_b_1938803.html [Accessed: 31 March 2021].

5. 'Discrimination at school: is a Black British history lesson repeating itself?', Lola Okolosie, *Guardian*, 15 November 2020. https://www.theguardian.com/education/2020/nov/15/discrimination-at-school-is-a-black-british-history-lesson-repeating-itself-small-axe-education-steve-mcqueen [Accessed: 31 March 2021].

28. My Father

1. Eke-Prince P.O. Ekwerekwu, *Know Onitsha Families* (Amakohson Printing Creation, 1989).

31. Professional, Personal Political

1. K. M. Hoffman, et al. (2016), 'Racial bias in pain assessment and treatment recommendations, and false beliefs about biological differences between blacks and whites', *Proceedings of the National Academy of Sciences of the United States of America*, 113 (16): 4296–430. https://www.pnas.org/content/113/16/4296 [Accessed: 31 March 2021].

32. The First UK Sickle Cell Nurse

1. L. Nyhagen Predelli et al., *Majority-Minority Relations in Contemporary Women's Movements: Strategic Sisterhood* (Palgrave Macmillan, 2012), p.55.
2. 'Colbert I. King', The History Makers, 4 May 2005. https://www.thehistorymakers.org/biography/colbert-i-king-40 [Accessed: 10 April 2021].
3. B. J. Culliton (1972), 'Sickle cell anemia: the route from obscurity to prominence', *Science*, 178: 138–142.
4. E. N. Anionwu and K. Atkin, *The Politics of Sickle Cell and Thalassaemia* (Open University Press, June 2001).

36. A Tough Role

1. E. N. Anionwu, 'Running a Sickle Cell Centre: Community Counselling' in J. K. Cruickshank and D. G. Beevers (eds.), *Ethnic Factors in Health and Disease* (Wright, 1989), pp.123–130.

Chapter 38: Forging Ahead

1. 'Overview: cystic fibrosis', NHS, ' undated. https://www.nhs.uk/conditions/cystic-fibrosis/ [Accessed: 2 April 2021].
2. Parliament UK, 'Memorandum by the NHS Sickle Cell and Thalassaemia Screening Programme (HI 86)', January 2008.

https://publications.parliament.uk/pa/cm200708/cmselect/cmhealth/422/422we238.htm [Accessed: 2 April 2021].

39. The Inspiring Mrs Mary Seacole

1. C. Staring-Derks et al. (2014), 'Mary Seacole: global nurse extraordinaire', *Journal of Advanced Nursing*, 71 (3): 514–25. https://www.uwl.ac.uk/sites/default/files/Academic-schools/College-of-Nursing-Midwifery-and-Healthcare/Web/PDF/Elizabeth%20Anionwu%20Papers/MarySeacole_jan%2010Nov2014.pdf [Accessed: 31 March 2021].
2. J. E. Gordon (1975), 'Mary Seacole: A forgotten nurse heroine of the Crimea', *Midwife, Health Visitor & Community Nurse*, 11 (2): 47–50.
3. C. Davis, 'Mary Seacole' New Statesman, (107, 39) 1984.
4. 'Decolonising Dermatology', Neil Singh, *Guardian*, 13 August 2020. https://www.theguardian.com/society/2020/aug/13/decolonising-dermatology-why-black-and-brown-skin-need-better-treatment [Accessed: 10 April 2021].

40. A Role Model

1. 'Churchill voted greatest Briton', BBC News, 24 November 2002. http://news.bbc.co.uk/1/hi/entertainment/2509465.stm [Accessed: 31 March 2021].
2. 100 Great Black Britons, undated. https://www.100great-blackbritons.com [Accessed: 31 March 2021].
3. J. Robinson, *Mary Seacole: The Charismatic Black Nurse Who Became a Heroine of the Crimea* (Robinson, 2006).
4. 'Mary Seacole statue', Mary Seacole Trust, undated. https://www.maryseacoletrust.org.uk/mary-seacole-statue/ [Accessed: 31 March 2021].
5. 'Betsi Cadwaladr', Chwarae Teg, undated. https://chwaraeteg.com/projects/wonderful-welsh-women/betsi-cadwaladr/ [Accessed: 10 April 2021]; N. R. Storey, *WRNS: The Women's Royal Naval Service* (Shire Publications, 2017), p.5; 'Mary

Francis Bridgeman', Wikipedia, undated. https://en.wikipedia.org/wiki/Mary_Francis_Bridgeman [Accessed: 10 April 2021]; 'Dasha from Sevastopol', Wikipedia, undated. https://en.wikipedia.org/wiki/Dasha_from_Sevastopol [Accessed: 10 April 2021].

41. Becoming Dame Elizabeth Nneka Anionwu

1. 'Just 3.5% of NHS trust chief nurses are from a BME background, data reveals', Healthcare Leader, 19 March 2019; https://healthcareleadernews.com/news/just-3-5-of-nhs-trust-chief-nurses-are-from-a-bme-background-data-reveals/ [Accessed: 31 March 2021].

42. Dreams from My Mother

1. 'Black people four times more likely to die from Covid-19, ONS finds', Robert Booth and Caelainn Barr, *Guardian*, 7 May 2020. https://www.theguardian.com/world/2020/may/07/black-people-four-times-more-likely-to-die-from-covid-19-ons-finds [Accessed: 31 March 2021]; 'Deaths of NHS staff from covid-19 analysed', Tim Cook, Emira Kursumovic and Simon Lennane, HSJ, 22 April 2020. https://www.hsj.co.uk/exclusive-deaths-of-nhs-staff-from-covid-19-analysed/7027471.article [Accessed: 31 March 2021].

2. 'Mary Agyapong: Pregnant nurse who died with Covid "felt pressured" to work', BBC News, 23 March 2021. https://www.bbc.co.uk/news/uk-england-beds-bucks-herts-56498978 [Accessed: 31 March 2021].

3. 'Rowena Arshad discusses contraception and controlling poor women's bodies', British Library, 15–16 June 2011. https://www.bl.uk/collection-items/rowena-arshad-contraception-and-controlling-poor-womens-bodies [Accessed: 31 March 2021].

4. 'Black women in the UK four times more likely to die in pregnancy or childbirth', Hannah Summers, *Guardian*, 15 January 2021. https://www.theguardian.com/global-devel-

opment/2021/jan/15/black-women-in-the-uk-four-times-more-likely-to-die-in-pregnancy-or-childbirth [Accessed: 31 March 2021]; 'Discrimination in mental health services', Mind, June 2019. https://www.mind.org.uk/news-campaigns/legal-news/legal-newsletter-june-2019/discrimination-in-mental-health-services/ [Accessed: 31 March 2021].

5. 'Death of sickle cell disease patient who rang 999 from hospital bed could have been prevented, coroner says', Matt Mathers, *Independent*, 8 April 2021. https://www.independent.co.uk/news/uk/home-news/evan-nathan-smith-death-sickle-cell-b1827443.html [Accessed: 9 April 2021].

6. 'How to Demand a Medical Breakthrough: Lessons from the AIDS Fight', Nurith Aizenman, NPR, 9 February 2019. https://www.npr.org/sections/health-shots/2019/02/09/689924838/how-to-demand-a-medical-breakthrough-lessons-from-the-aids-fight?t=1617209125893 [Accessed: 31 March 2021].

7. 'Member of Royal family worried about colour of Archie's skin, says Meghan, Duchess of Sussex', *Telegraph*, 8 March 2021. https://www.telegraph.co.uk/royal-family/2021/03/08/meghan-duchess-sussex-says-member-royal-family-worried-son-archies/ [Accessed: 31 March 2021].